PRAISE FOR

*Passion & Presence*

"Learn to inhabit your living body with sacred presence. This is a wonderful guide to deepening intimacy through the seasons of our loving relationships."

> —TARA BRACH
> author of *Radical Compassion* and *Radical Acceptance*

"This book brings real tools to all couples looking to increase the passion and connection in their relationship, whatever stage they find themselves. Anyone looking at this book will find a new way to be present with their partner."

> —TAMMY NELSON, PHD
> author of *Getting the Sex You Want*

"In this hopeful and radically transformative book, Maci Daye takes us into the under-layers that block our true sexual potential and outlines a path out of resignation to joyful pleasure. The surprising secret to sustaining or reigniting passion between long-term lovers begins within, and our capacity to 'be here' versus 'get off' is vital."

> —CHELSEA WAKEFIELD, PHD, LCSW
> author of *In Search of Aphrodite*

"In this comprehensive and practical book, Maci Daye shares hard-earned wisdom from decades of helping couples use their sexual issues as paths to becoming more fully alive, intimate, and erotic. She writes that 'Great sex is a mind-set, not a skill-set,' and proves that with a host of engaging case-studies and experiential exercises that will help you find and heal the inner obstacles to great sex."

—RICHARD SCHWARTZ, PHD
creator of the Internal Family Systems model of psychotherapy

"Maci Daye brings her decades of experience and her wide-open heart to this gentle and wise book. On these pages, you are invited into deeper connection—with your partner and with yourself. Your sexual healing starts now!"

—ALEXANDRA SOLOMON, PHD
author of *Loving Bravely* and *Taking Sexy Back*

"In this beautiful book, Maci Daye explores the physical, emotional, psychological, and spiritual dimensions of sexuality. If you are looking for a quick fix to your bedroom boredom, this is not for you. And to that, I say hallelujah, because there are no handy short cuts around sensual disconnect, no easy way to break out of the familiarity trance and bring mindful aliveness to this moment, this touch, this kiss. But if you want to know what it means to be truly naked, together, I strongly recommend *Passion and Presence*."

—CHERYL FRASER, PHD
author of *Buddha's Bedroom*, creator of *Become Passion: An Online Course for Couples*

# Passion & Presence

## A COUPLE'S GUIDE

to Awakened Intimacy and Mindful Sex

## MACI DAYE

SHAMBHALA

Shambhala Publications, Inc.
4720 Walnut Street
Boulder, Colorado 80301
www.shambhala.com

"Figure 6.2, Plane of Possibility Map" is from *The Mindful Therapist: A Clinician's Guide to Mindsight and Neural Integration* by Daniel J. Siegel. Copyright ©2010 by Mind Your Brain, Inc. Used by permission of W. W. Norton & Company, Inc.

Cover art: Vera Lair/Stocksy
Cover design: Amanda Weiss
Interior design: Kate Huber-Parker

9 8 7 6 5 4 3 2 1

First Edition
Printed in the United States of America

♾ This edition is printed on acid-free paper that meets the American National Standards Institute Z39.48 Standard.
♾ This book is printed on 30% postconsumer recycled paper.
For more information please visit www.shambhala.com.
Shambhala Publications is distributed worldwide by Penguin Random House, Inc., and its subsidiaries.

Library of Congress Cataloging-in-Publication Data
Names: Daye, Maci, author.
Title: Passion and presence: a couple's guide to awakened intimacy and mindful sex / Maci Daye.
Description: First edition. | Boulder, Colorado: Shambhala, [2020] | Includes bibliographical references and index.
Identifiers: LCCN 2020003116 | ISBN 9781611808131 (paperback; alk. paper)
Subjects: LCSH: Sex instruction. | Intimacy (Psychology) | Mindfulness (Psychology)
Classification: LCC HQ31 .D29 2020 | DDC 158.2—dc23
LC record available at https://lccn.loc.gov/2020003116

# Contents

List of Exercises    ix
Introduction    1

1 • AWAKENED INTIMACY
The Journey of Conscious Erotic Coupling    9

2 • EROTIC PRESENCE
Cultivating a State of Mind for
Intimate and Creative Sex    33

3 • EROTIC COOPERATION
Holding Hands through the Hard Stuff    61

4 • EROTIC TRANSFORMATION
Healing and Growing through Sex    95

5 • EROTIC EXPRESSION
Overcoming Shame to Reclaim Your Full Self    129

6 • EROTIC ATTUNEMENT
Dancing with Eros from the Inside Out    161

7 • EROTIC SUSTENANCE
   Tending Our Magic through the Seasons   189

Acknowledgments   217
Glossary   223
Notes   225
Index   249
About the Author   261

# List of Exercises

1. AWAKENED INTIMACY
Noticing Our Reactions to Having Goal-Free Sex    30

2. EROTIC PRESENCE
Seeing Fresh    56
Mindful Touch    58

3. EROTIC COOPERATION
Getting to Know Your Protector and Protected Parts    89

4. EROTIC TRANSFORMATION
Mindful Self-Study    126
Planting a Heart    127

5. EROTIC EXPRESSION
Experiencing the Creative Potential of Parts Play    155

6. EROTIC ATTUNEMENT
Moving Mindfully through the EROS Cycle    188

7. EROTIC SUSTENANCE
Crafting Our Sustenance Plan    215

# Introduction

Pam and Stu are sitting on floor cushions looking excited and nervous. We are in a private conference during one of my Passion and Presence[1] couples retreats. After exchanging pleasantries, they tell me why they are here. Pam is soft-spoken and has a kind face. She explains that three children, a relocation, and a battle with breast cancer killed her sex drive. "I was weak and depressed," Pam says. "Stuart knew I wasn't up for sex, so he backed off."

Stuart, a sincere-looking man in his mid-forties, is quick to own his part: "I felt so helpless when I saw Pam suffering like that. I was trying to be strong for us, but in bed, my fear took over, I guess." He hesitates, "Sometimes, I still can't perform." Pam touches Stu's arm with so much tenderness, my eyes well. "We were both so tired," says Pam, continuing with the story, "that eventually we stopped having sex. Now that I've gotten a clean bill of health, we're hoping to get our groove back." She laughs shyly and shoots Stu an encouraging look.

Pam and Stu are describing what I call a stage 2 relationship to a tee. At stage 1 of their relationship, they could idle in bed riding waves of passion. However, children, a health crisis, and real-life responsibilities punctured their erotic bubble. For the past nineteen years, they have faced constant change and boatloads of uncertainty. Real life is complicated, and so is real-life sex.

Like Pam and Stu, the couples that come to my retreats want to deepen or restore their erotic connection. Although some are still in the blush of new love, the vast majority attends because routine or even absence has replaced the smooth and rewarding sex they once had. Sex has become fraught with complications that seem too hard to resolve on their own.

There are also some couples at the retreats that have never experienced fireworks in bed. For them, sex was bumpy or passionless right from the start. They hanker for something they have never actually tasted, at least not with each other. About a quarter of these couples bring a history of trauma with them. One or both partners find sex aversive or have associated routine sex with safety. They attend the retreats because avoidance and routines are robbing both themselves and their relationship of vibrancy.

What unites most of the couples that attend the retreats is that they don't know how to "change" the unsatisfying status quo of their erotic lives together. They want to experience erotic vitality, but their efforts have thus far failed to get them what they want.

Myriad forces ensure that we falter at stage 2 of our erotic journey. Unfortunately, with no more preparation for this stage than any other, we are forced to rely on our wits to navigate this steep and often de-eroticizing pass. Regrettably, the evidence shows that for Pam and Stu and many others, "winging it" isn't working. At last count, 20 million American couples were in sexless marriages, and 50 percent of sexually active couples were unhappy with the amount or kind of sex they were having.[2]

Walter and Ingrid, another couple at the retreat, bring an air of tension into the interview room. "We've tried *everything*, and we still rarely have sex," bemoans Walter, somewhat bitterly. "We've even gone to a swingers club!" confirms Ingrid. She studies my face for praise or reprimand. Seeing none, she continues: "But, I'm tired," she says weakly. "Maybe we should give it a rest for a while?" Her question sounds more like a plea.

I see Ingrid's point. She and Walter are part of a growing class of "sexual warriors" who are taking up arms to fight their declining drive. In the past two years, they've tried Tantra, light bondage, and the extended orgasm technique to keep passion burning. Sadly, despite their efforts to be skillful and adventurous lovers, they still struggle in bed.

Rather than focusing on new thrills, techniques, or positions, what really sparks awakened intimacy is a mindful approach. It works with your *consciousness*, not your behavior. A mindful approach isn't about trying to overcome anything; it doesn't take the view that there is something "wrong" that has to be "fixed"—at least not with force. Committed sex is complicated and will continue to be so as we age, face ongoing stressors, and deal with overfamiliarity.

Given this complexity, *can we stay erotically alive in a long-term relationship?*

Often, couples are encouraged to add novelty to spice things up. This prescription usually involves much doing, such as learning new positions, dressing up and changing our appearance, or purchasing props and toys. In their attempts to add novelty, many of the couples I see, like Walter and Ingrid, are already working *too* hard. As a result, sex has become a production, rather than the respite that they seek.

We need an alternative to this *doing* bias which dominates much of sex therapy as well as self-help books and magazines. The answer is mindfulness practice. Mindfulness—awareness of the present moment— engenders an open and curious mind-state that allows us to relate to any encounter as if for the first time. Mindfulness can help couples experience novelty as a *continuous* feature of their sexual encounters, rather than relying on new techniques to heat things up in bed.

When we are curious and exploratory, it is possible to access the "novelty state," which is outside the limiting scripts or fixed ideas that shape our sexual encounters. To access this state, we have to train our attention—thus the emphasis on mindfulness practice—otherwise, we will bring the same automatic behaviors to every encounter.

The dulling of passion, although a challenge, also provides an opportunity to usher couples like Walter and Ingrid across a new erotic threshold. Searching outside for more skill, sensation, and variety is deafening and exhausting. It is also pointing them in the wrong direction. Like a navigation system, eros broadcasts signals through the body. Sex can be a wakeful adventure when we let eros lead. However, to hear these signals, we must be present and embodied.

This radical approach to eros requires a shift—from an outside-in orientation to an inside-out orientation. The inside-out approach can also help us discover what is shutting down our aliveness. Reviving and maintaining sexual vitality is a path of practice that involves developing new skills. My popular retreat series, Passion and Presence, helps couples hone this skill set—and this book brings these skills to you.

For many years I have shared Passion and Presence in the United States, Mexico, Australia, and Europe with my husband Halko Weiss. Like all couples, we have struggled with age-related changes, bewildering stressors, and overfamiliarity. We have also felt the painful effects of our early learning when sex-negative imprints from our pasts have climbed into bed with us. Fortunately, we have become more connected and sexually expressed by using the very same tools I share in this book. These tools come from a range of sources, including Hakomi Mindful Somatic Psychotherapy, neuroscience, sex therapy, trauma therapy, and systems theory. My training in these areas has helped me understand why sex becomes complicated when the novelty wears off and why almost all couples struggle to stay erotically connected.

In every retreat I lead, there is a moment where the energy of the group shifts. At the beginning, people are reluctant to speak openly about their sexual difficulties. A few hours in, awkward silences give way to smiles of recognition, vigorous head nods, and unsolicited disclosures. My heart always swells when the first wall comes down. By sharing instead of hiding our real-life experiences, we rid ourselves of the shame we carry that we alone are broken or abnormal.

Sitting in circles with couples of different backgrounds, orientations, and ages has shown me that passionate sex is rare in long-term relationships. Many couples report that the real-life sex they are having is more often triggering or routine. They feel deadened, inadequate, and lonely. I hear the same things in my sex therapy practice. Jerome and Keisha miss the magic they once made in the bedroom. Abbey and Quinn insist they have incompatible sexual styles. He wants to "get to it," says Abbey, who longs for more time to connect as a couple. Quinn complains that Abbey's "slow warm-up" and need to talk before they make love interrupts his flow. Riya is afraid of being overwhelmed by sex, and Nalini becomes guilt-ridden when she and Riya make love.

If you're in a long-term relationship, you've probably experienced one or more of these issues. You may even wonder if your journey as a romantic couple has ended. Like Jerome and Keisha, you may want more sizzle in your sex life. Like Abby and Quinn, you may believe you and your partner are sexually incompatible. Maybe, like Riya and Nalini, you think sex is a good thing, *in principle*, but are maligned by unpleasant feelings when you have it.

In the West, we tend to view these problems as impediments to sex and try to fix them. The Eastern philosophies of Buddhism and Taoism avow that life includes *both* joy *and* suffering. Such a perspective makes room for the difficult, even confronting feelings that sometimes arise when we have sex. A core message of Passion and Presence is that mature love—meaning love that endures beyond the intoxicating, highly libidinous first six to twenty-four months—is fraught with complexity. Many books focus on the "joy of sex," to the exclusion of the real pains that are part of our real-life sex lives.

In contrast, a mindful mind-set recognizes that life, and therefore sex, is a package deal. Passion and Presence embraces this both/and perspective. It offers a way to orient to sex that derives from the Eastern wisdom traditions and somatic psychology. These streams suggest a path of *being* rather than doing. They encourage us to look inward and to allow, instead of forcing anything or striving to reach a goal.

The both/and approach means that this book explores not only the benefits of mindful intimacy, but also barriers to pleasure and sexual expression. "When you stand in the light of a close relationship, you must learn to deal with the shadow," write Gay and Kathlyn Hendricks.[3] Sex illuminates our shadows, which makes it both triggering and full of growth potential. Most people honestly don't know why they have roadblocks to sex. Unfortunately, open communication, a vacation, or lingerie won't shed light on their shadows, but mindful sex will. We can use the illuminating power of eros for healing.

When early imprints light up during sex, we can feel very naked. However, this nakedness allows us to see what holds us back from experiencing our full aliveness. Sexual triggers are often trailheads to shame marks and erotic wounds that are ready to heal. Because Passion and Presence is relational, embodied, and goal-free, many people with a trauma history respond to it favorably. However, everyone who has grown up in a sex-negative culture can benefit from the healing in this approach.

A central premise of Passion and Presence is that our early learning gets in under the radar and becomes the basis of our internal models of sex. These models shape our behaviors in bed automatically and generate emotional reactions for *all of us*. The mindful approach to intimacy involves investigating these reactions with compassion and curiosity.

Does this mean we need to give up thinking of sex as fun, nurturing, or naughty? Certainly not. The both/and approach gives equal weight to the pleasure side of the sexual equation. Eros plays through all the keys—major and minor—and we can enjoy the spontaneous intermingling of our eros energies in surprising and delightful ways too. The more embodied we become, the better able we are to attune to our eros energy and experience the deeply sensual, pleasurable, and regenerative qualities of sex.

Passion and Presence shares a three-stage model that shows how to move from unconscious to conscious erotic coupling. Each chapter explores ideas and stories in depth, then offers reflections and exercises for you to try alone or with your partner to deepen your experience. The stories are composite cases of the many couples I have worked with in my workshops and therapy. I have changed the names, ages, and other identifying information to ensure confidentiality. However, the issues presented in these cases emerge so often in my sessions with couples that I have come to regard them as common themes of "real-life" sex.

Chapter 1, "Awakened Intimacy," describes how all couples move from enchantment (stage 1) to disenchantment (stage 2) with time. When passion tarnishes, many couples disengage or source aliveness elsewhere. At stage 3, re-enchantment, couples wake up by working through their issues as a mindful team. They discover the real magic of mindful sex lies in cultivating a curious and open mind. When we allow eros to lead us, sex can be transformative.

Chapter 2, "Erotic Presence," looks at how you can change your mind-set to recover the curiosity, creativity, and magic that makes sex a wakeful adventure. Many stage 2 couples approach sex as a chore or a performance test. They engage in lifeless, predictable routines that are efficient but uninspiring. Here you will see how stage 3 couples wake up from automaticity.

The process of befriending, exploring, and ultimately transforming blocks to erotic expression requires a deep and abiding couple alliance. In chapter 3, "Erotic Cooperation," you will learn how to nurture your connection to become more compassionate and loving. You will gain a skill set to work with feelings that arise when you get emotionally naked together that will help you "hold hands through the hard stuff."

Healing wounds rendered visible by sex is the crux of chapter 4, "Erotic Transformation." You will learn how to shift from lovemaking to emotional repair and back again, reframing challenges as opportunities for healing, rather than obstacles to sex. I share a simple technique for working with triggers on the spot and show you how to detach "now from then" in cases of trauma.

"Naked" sex involves more than taking off your clothes. It requires showing different parts of yourselves and sharing your hidden desires. In chapter 5, "Erotic Expression," we look at creative ways to express parts that may have been long sealed off by shame and adult responsibilities. Too much safety can stifle growth and shrink your erotic playground to one small sandbox. I will help you create a relational container in which it becomes safe to expand as you use your erotic portal to release shame.

Letting go of your routines and embracing uncertainty enables you to reach higher levels of creativity through collaborative emergence. In chapter 6, "Erotic Attunement," you will use your felt sense to follow the flow of eros energy unfolding within and between you.

Chapter 7, "Erotic Sustenance," discusses how to have a vital erotic life into your "golden years," remaining enchanted by expanding your vision of sex even as function declines. By tending eros as a couple, you can ensure the magic endures and that your sex life remains nourishing and fruitful throughout your journey together.

*Passion and Presence* offers numerous ways to transform barriers to intimacy as a couple. You can experience more play, engagement, and creative expression, no matter how stuck you feel right now or how long you've been together. Whether your goal is enrichment or healing, here you will find a peaceful path to passionate sex and a wakeful and undefended way of loving. Along the way, you will meet other couples that have opened the padlocks to pleasure and accessed their erotic potential by embracing this curious and adventurous path. These gifts are waiting for you. Welcome to the circle.

# 1.

# AWAKENED INTIMACY

## The Journey of Conscious Erotic Coupling

To be in love is merely to be in a state of perpetual anesthesia—to mistake an ordinary young man for a Greek god or an ordinary young woman for a goddess.
—H. L. MENCKEN[1]

Anyone who has experienced the pull of enchantment knows it is both exhilarating and wrenching to the body and mind. When Cupid's golden arrow first strikes us, we can't sleep, focus, or eat until we reunite with our beloved. Our sexual and romantic fixations are often intrusive and relentless. In a full-blown infatuation, nothing else can get our attention in quite the same way. For the vast majority, sex at this stage is dazzling, and our drive to have it is irrepressible as well.

Most of us don't know or forget that what comes next is the prick of Cupid's second arrow, made of lead. When the leaden arrow pierces our state of rapture, our desire cools, possibly to indifference or even aversion. Now sex may deliver more disappointment than dopamine. Where has the object of our infatuation gone? Many starry-eyed lovers feel duped when the deity they have fallen for turns out to be merely a mortal under this harsh and glaring light.

We all pine for love, and feel the excitement of believing we have found it in our new beloved. Thus, when our relationship fails to live up to its early promise of everlasting passion, we feel despondent. We might hope that an exciting holiday or a sex workshop will rekindle enchantment, but the remedy for Cupid's leaden arrow is not a quick fix. Conversely, we may believe that only a sword can sever us from the Gordian knot of our tangled disappointments, but a complete severance is not always the answer either.

Of course, many couples resign themselves to what they consider to be fate. They let disappointment settle into the relationship, so that routine and predictability take root. This phase of disenchantment is when couples often attend one of my Passion and Presence retreats. Participants are relieved to discover there is an alternative to total severance or resignation. When we realize that Cupid's leaden arrow inevitably follows the golden arrow, it is possible to adopt a different understanding of our relationship's purpose and forge a new erotic path.

This book is about the path to revitalizing, renewing, and restoring your erotic connection no matter your age or years together. I call this the "naked path." It is *naked* because it is related to sex, which feels vulnerable and exposing to many people, and also because our early wounds and limiting beliefs become visible to ourselves when we are sexual with a long-term partner. It is a *path* because it has three stages and points us in a direction as a couple.

The naked path, like any established path, has a well-drawn map of the terrain, highlighting potential obstacles and dangers. Together we will explore the kinds of obstacles many couples face in a committed relationship. As your guide, I will give you a tool kit to navigate these barriers and point out guideposts to help you find your way to re-enchantment. We will dig into questions that occupy therapists and scientists alike: Why does desire plummet with familiarity, and why is sex with our partner so complicated?

Although many of us want to rush the process, becoming a conscious couple is a developmental journey. We move from a state of fusion, which makes stage 1 so exciting and consuming, to fashioning an independent and erotically attuned self within the relationship at stage 3. Along the way, we inevitably pass through trials and disappointments that can strengthen us as a couple or tear us apart. For this reason, the naked path is also like a challenging physical expedition. We discover beliefs and habits that block our confidence in our erotic creativity while experiencing the exhilaration of triumphing even when things feel at their most hopeless.

## LOVE AND SEX THROUGH THE STAGES

### Stage 1: Erotic Enchantment

The first few months of courtship I call "erotic enchantment" because we are literally under a spell. A cocktail of endogenous opioids, mixed with a splash of dopamine, the bonding hormone oxytocin, and lust-inducing testosterone spikes our desire. This biochemical cocktail is responsible for the blissed-out, turned-on feelings that we more than likely attribute to our partner being "right" for us.[2]

At stage 1, enchantment, we sing in perfect unison. In this melodic interlude, we also experience a sense of safety and trust. We open our heart to receive love and in return, become more loving ourselves. In our "love state," we are patient, flexible, and generous. Seemingly immune to the setbacks and inconveniences of everyday life, we tolerate rude drivers, lateness, and pesky colleagues. We can even operate on a deficit of sleep without feeling cranky or daft.

This heady combination of euphoria, openness, and swagger can cause stage 1 couples to overrate their forecasting abilities, especially with regard to sex. They naively assume that the frequent and disinhibited sex they are having now will continue into their problem-free futures. It doesn't. The passion cocktail is merely nature's trick to get us ready for the next task: procreation.

Gay, straight, in-between, or beyond, we all come equipped with the same evolutionary hardware. However, to our animal brain, the chase is much more thrilling than keeping what we capture.[3] In other words, dating is a far greater turn-on than lying next to each other night after night. The mystery, longing, uncertainty, and novelty—all fodder for hot Hollywood sex—goes missing when we bed down with an "always available" mate.

## STRESSED AND SEXLESS

Many factors can contribute to the absence of sex in committed relationships, but chief among them is our mounting to-do lists. Enchanted couples want to spend as much time as possible together, preferably in bed. Between the sheets, they travel without a map because they aren't trying to get anywhere. Their sexual behaviors are entirely unscripted; this is what makes sex at stage 1 exciting and mysterious. However, when Cupid's leaden arrow stings, our attention now goes toward real-world responsibilities. We lose our unfettered curiosity to sexual routines, and we privilege efficiency over exploration.

At stage 2, disenchantment, we usually have to cross a divide of chores, caretaking, and work to find each other. For many couples, building that bridge turns into another duty that comes to feel like too much work. Moreover, the growing gap between the demands of our lives and our capacity to meet them keeps many of us chronically tense and stressed. We are literally "in over our heads," claims Robert Kegan, a leading developmental psychologist.[4] We may be smart, but our brains have not kept stride with the bewildering array of modern-day problems we ask them to solve.

This impossibility doesn't stop us from trying! Feeling overwhelmed and inept, we are apt to speed up even more. Supersonic speed is efficient, but terrible for sex. It dulls our pleasure receptors and dampens our signals of arousal. When and if we have sex, we often settle for the fast-food version—gulping down something quick and easy instead of pausing, slowing down and noticing what we truly hunger for.

Running full tilt to get to the end zone robs partner sex of the excitement and mystery that leads unhurried lovers to unexpectedly rich places. To discover the hidden gems that dwell in the side streets and alleyways of our erotic imagination, we have to ditch our watches and how-to books. Doing so demands nothing less than a radical reenvisioning of sex from a goal-oriented achievement to a live and connected experience. In other words, it has to be worth showing up for sex.

Unfortunately, the pressure to "Look good," "Do it right," or thinking we have to "Want it all the time," converts sex into yet another demand. Gripped by the resulting performance pressure, we concoct legitimate-sounding excuses, such as lack of time, energy, or privacy, to mask our growing sexual anxiety. Sadly, the absence of quality of sex provides only more evidence that it is we who are lacking when it comes to experiencing "great sex."

This state of anxious mobilization inhibits eros, particularly in women who tend to be multitaskers. Stress creates vascular constriction, leading to low libido; and in extreme cases, sexual dysfunction.[5] With less testosterone than men, most women need to power down their nervous system to feel ready and possibly safe enough for sex.[6]

Moreover, as we progress from romance to commitment, we become victims of a biochemical bait and switch. The hormones that engender feelings of attachment—principally oxytocin and vasopressin—supplant the hormones that make us lust for one another at stage 1.[7] While emotional attachment keeps us in long-term relationships, it does nothing to fire up our loins.[8] However, most self-help approaches emphasize performance to stoke the flames again, which can lead to what I call the "novelty trap."

## THE NOVELTY TRAP

Stage 1 couples are awash in anticipation and excitement because everything is new. Novelty, defined by the *Cambridge English Dictionary* as "something that has not been experienced before and so is interesting," abounds. Novelty is, indisputably, a powerful attention grabber. We notice music in our surrounds when we hear it for the first time, but the same piece fades into the periphery of awareness when played over and over. A delightful new dish becomes unremarkable when served at every meal. Likewise, a sizzling sex life grows stale when we repeat the same moves in bed with our partner every time.

After some years together, even couples with the hots for each other long to change up the menu. Some couples adventure outside of their relationship to recover novelty. Those who prefer monogamy to what sex-advice columnist Dan Savage calls "monogamish" are often advised to add variety to their lovemaking.[9] I call this approach the "novelty prescription."

When curiosity ebbs at stage 2, we try to lasso our short attention spans by *doing* new things.

Here is a list of some recommendations for recovering novelty I have seen over the years:

Scour adult stores for props and toys
Learn new positions
Make love at different times and in different places
Incorporate role-play
Wear costumes and lingerie
Go on vacation
Talk dirty
Share fantasies
Read erotica or watch porn together

All of these activities can be playful additions to your erotic treasure trove; however, the novelty prescription has essential drawbacks. First, it implies that novelty is a spice we source "out there." While we may experience an uptick in desire from one of these recommendations, it is likely to be a mere flash in the pan. What's more, these activities require time, energy, and money—the very resources depleted couples often lack. Worse, the novelty prescription can become a trap that leads to even more erotic absence. That is, in the search for new thrills, we may disconnect from our embodied eroticism, which, as we shall see, is the source of re-enchantment.

Novelty comes in two dimensions: wide and deep. We can focus on what we do and add new things to our sex life to create novelty (wide)—as we saw in the novelty prescriptions above. Alternatively, we can learn to pay attention again (deep). The deep route requires training our attention to be present with the moment to notice things we miss when we are fast, automatic, or focused outside of ourselves.

Paying attention enables us to discover new things in familiar places. For instance, we can notice aspects of the scenery we ordinarily miss on our harried drive to work. Sexually, we feel and sense more deeply if we are *just there* and then let our eros energy lead us somewhere new. Just as music has different melodies, tempos, and dynamics, so does the eros energy that moves inside of you. Rather than adding novelty to spice up your sex life, here you will begin to see yourself as an instrument through which this energy plays.

Eros energy constantly shape-shifts and blends with our changing physical energy and mood. How you relate to this variability has everything to do with how you judge your sex life. If you see change—especially when it is a downward movement—as a problem to overcome, then you may remain disenchanted. If you can accept the natural fluctuating peaks and troughs of eros energy, then you can have a rewarding sexual relationship for many years to come.

## DISCOVERING YOUR PURE EROTIC POTENTIAL

Make an empty space in any corner of your mind and creativity will instantly fill it.
—Dee Hock[10]

When we relinquish goals and set courses, eros can go in any direction. While we can never delete our memory bank entirely, we can aspire to bring freshness and uniqueness to our lovemaking. Creativity—as opposed to novelty—in the bedroom isn't necessarily about trying something new or kinky. Creativity comes when each time we can imagine this is the first and only time with our partner.

While having sex, we try to establish an "anything is possible" state of mind, which is simple but not easy to attain. If we are present to the moment, to ourselves, and to our partner, we can discover that we have unlimited creative potential. I call this erotic creativity pure erotic potential (or PEP), which is something we can experience with mindfulness.

Although pure erotic potential sounds like something to work toward, we don't have to strain or make an effort to reach our PEP. We access our PEP by becoming present, curious, and exploratory rather than goal-directed. As a result, we can experience every encounter as fresh and new, no matter how long we have been together.

We do not have to be "good in bed" to access our PEP, either; we merely engage freely and openly with the erotic energy unfolding between us. However, because of past wounds, habits, and expectations, we have developed barriers to our PEP. These barriers generally emerge at stage 2 of our relationship, when the intensity of our desire ebbs in response to changes in biochemistry, external demands, and sexual familiarity.

This book is about learning to access your PEP, individually, and as a couple. Separately, you are each responsible for looking at your mindset concerning sex. Exercises and reflections will help you explore how past experiences, beliefs, or attitudes are inhibiting you from accessing your eros energy. Together, it is about becoming a mindful team. I will encourage you to undertake activities that make mindfulness a key component of your sexual life.

Instead of trying to fix yourselves, you will cultivate curiosity about the barriers that are limiting you from being fully self-expressed. A mindful approach is a path and practice rather than a solution. It is about creating a conscious erotic coupling that enables you to become more resilient, compassionate, and engaged as a couple.

## Stage 2: Erotic Disenchantment

Thou blind fool love, what dost thou to mine eyes
That they behold and see not what they see?
—Shakespeare[11]

While our stage 1 Bacchanalian lovefest is fun and exciting, it is also short-lived. We cannot live in what appeared to be a state of perfect harmony forever. The passage from childhood to adulthood moves from a symbiotic fusion to separation and differentiation.[12] So does the passage to erotic maturity.

At the beginning of a romantic relationship, our boundaries are permeable, and we merge sexually and emotionally. While the intimate bubble we form with our new partner is initially comforting, if we stay there too long, we will die from a lack of oxygen. Like a firefly in a glass jar, the light diminishes until it goes out of our relationship entirely.

Where once we were starstruck, now, in stage 2, we've succumbed to one or more of the three main erotic tribulations: feeling lonely, mad, or bored. Alone because we have lost our "twin"; mad for being tricked; and, bored if we decide there will be no more magic. For when the love drugs wear off at stage 2, our different sexual rhythms, appetites, and callings appear to be enormous and fundamentally incompatible.

Here are a few examples I have heard from stage 2 couples in the counseling room:

I'm horny all the time; you never want sex.
I'm a morning person; you're a night person.
I like tender stroking; you like spanking.
I want to make love; you want to get off.
I want to change it up; you like how it is.
I like anal play. Yuck!

As the proverb goes, "Marriage is when two people become as one; the trouble starts when they try to decide which one."[13] Take, as an example, Abbey and Quinn. The couple met four years earlier at a mutual friend's thirty-second birthday party. Both describe their initial attraction as "electrifying." Quinn found Abbey easy to talk to and was put at ease by her disarming smile. Abbey found Quinn to be an engaging listener and was captivated by his sensitivity and charm. Over drinks the following night, Abbey learned that Quinn was an outdoors enthusiast who volunteered at a local animal shelter. Abbey was a financial consultant who dreamed of becoming a baker.

When they had sex a week later, they idled in bed for hours, exploring fjords of pleasure previously unknown to either. Abbey described Quinn's lovemaking as "sensuous, hot, and deeply in tune." Quinn described Abbey as adventurous and spirited in bed. Their relationship seemed to bring out the best in them. Quinn felt fun and spontaneous around Abbey. Abbey felt peaceful and alluring. Finally, it seemed, they had both met "The One."

Eight months later, Abbey and Quinn moved in together. However, after another eight months of "conjugal bliss," they began to quarrel. One day it was about whose family to visit over the holidays, the next, which restaurant to go to or whose turn it was to clean out the kitty litter. At first, they recovered quickly from these rows, but over time, their arguments grew more heated. It was the opposite of their rapidly cooling sex life. When they had sex, which was now hardly ever, it was as if a riptide had swept these once synchronous swimmers apart. They lost their grace and perfect timing, and all of their moves felt "off."

Abbey and Quinn had been, in each other's eyes, card-carrying members of the Hellenic pantheon. Now the fallen Olympians were sitting on opposite ends of my couch, tossing blame back and forth. "All you want is sex!" Abbey charges. "Well, you used to want sex as much as I do," counters Quinn. Abbey's retort is teary, "That's because I felt you wanted *me*; now, I could be anyone lying there." "How can you say that? You're the one I want, but you won't let me get close to you," Quinn says, sounding exasperated. They grow quiet before turning to me. "Maybe we don't love each other anymore," wonders Quinn aloud. "Or, never did!" accuses Abbey. "Maybe we jumped in too soon," he acquiesces, "before we knew each other. We might have realized that we're not right for each other and spared ourselves a lot of pain."

Like many couples, Abbey and Quinn expected sex to be as it was in that first phase of enchantment before they moved in together. They didn't know that committed sex is complicated because it is naked—both emotionally and erotically. For this reason, nearly every couple will eventually experience sexual difficulties of one kind or another. It doesn't matter how sexy you are, how well you perform, or how much you do or once loved your partner.

Of course, many theories try to account for our plummeting desire in a committed relationship. Some paint broad strokes related to evolutionary biology, mainly, whether humans are fit for monogamy. Others blame orgasm-centered sex for triggering a cascade of mood-dampening biochemicals that can lead to depression, irritability, boredom, and fatigue.[14] Still, others attribute flagging libido to "overfamiliarity," which refers to the numbing effect of habituation and the de-eroticizing impact of too much closeness.

In turn, each theory proposes a cure. We are urged by some experts to become more skillful or adventurous lovers, as in the novelty prescription above. Others advocate for multiple partners, slow sex, or ejaculatory control. Still, others suggest trying to trick the brain into producing the chemicals of desire by introducing naughtiness into our companionate union. While these approaches have value, many couples who end up in my consulting room have tried these strategies to no avail. Why is this so?

In my experience, few of these remedies address the emotional dynamics that make even the best and most beautiful lovers withdraw from sex in a committed relationship. At stage 2, you have to deal with the fact that you are now navigating a phase of increasing complexity without the rush of excitement that characterizes stage 1. On top of this, when passion fades, and the pressures of everyday life take over, limiting beliefs and old wounds reveal themselves, and sex can trigger unpleasant feelings. Such nakedness can be confronting, if not threatening, to a relationship.

Insecurities that were silenced by the blinding enchantment of stage 1 often reappear with a vengeance at stage 2. Not uncommonly, they play out in the bedroom, as was the case for Abbey, who grew up in a shame-based home. Quinn's family pushed conflict under the rug. Consequently, he never learned how to express his emotions skillfully and is unequipped to handle Abbey's. As happens so often at stage 2, each partner blames the other for their growing disenchantment. Not knowing it is possible to join forces to address their problems as a team, Abbey and Quinn felt stuck and hopeless about their relationship.

When we understand the devastating but inevitable sting of Cupid's leaden arrow, we can see it for what it is: namely, a catalyst for growth. When the covers come off, as they do at stage 2, we can use that nakedness to turn things around. Sex can become the means to "smoke out" the issues buried inside of us—limiting beliefs, imprints, and wounds—that stifle our erotic aliveness. This idea is at the heart of the naked path.

As we shall see, there are many barriers to our PEP that can be a buzzkill in the bedroom, including early imprints about yourself, others, and not the least of all—sex. However, our relationship story does not have to end here at stage 2. We can instead take the naked path to stage 3, which I call erotic re-enchantment. The rest of this book will show you how to get there.

## Stage 3: Erotic Re-enchantment

Perhaps, like Quinn, you feel like you are drowning in the disenchantment of stage 2. Maybe you believe the magic has left your relationship for good. If so, it may comfort you to know that disenchantment is a mile marker on the road to conscious erotic love. The proverbial "bubble burst" at stage 2 is painful, to be sure. It may also be a sign that you are ready to do the work to grow without sacrificing your erotic vitality.

While at stage 1, we felt expansive both sexually and emotionally, this peak experience was only temporary. Staying enchanted *consciously*—not blindly, as is the case in stage 1—is the intent of stage 3 coupling. As the African proverb says, "Smooth seas do not make skillful sailors." We can say the same for lovers. We have to journey through stage 2 and the valleys of a committed relationship to reach that summit consciously. Doing so takes work and a commitment to privileging growth over comfort.

Arriving at stage 3 is not a function of time and familiarity. You may be in a relatively new coupling or a relationship of many decades. In either case, the re-enchantment of stage 3 involves seeing difficulties as an erotic portal to growth. Growth means that we choose to "wake up" together as we work through our erotic challenges as a team.

I hope that you can hear the good news in what I am saying: re-enchantment is possible. Together you both can reignite the erotic flame of your relationship. A mindful approach, which is the cornerstone of Passion and Presence, gives us the sky view. When we can see that we are stuck in old patterns and beliefs we can begin to come into the present, which is necessary to heal and transform.

A mindful approach breeds acceptance of "real-life" sex and cultivates stores of compassion for our partner and our self. As Anaïs Nin explains: "Where the myth fails, human love begins. Then we love a human being, not our dream, but a human being with flaws."[15] At stage 3, we let go of ideas that we should be flawless or strive for perfect pitch. We understand our partner has wishes that are different from but as honorable as our own. Moreover, our differences stretch us to go further on the naked path than we would travel on our own.

## THE NAKED PATH TO AWAKENED INTIMACY

Instead of looking to a relationship for shelter, we could welcome its power to wake us up in those areas where we are asleep and where we avoid naked, direct contact with life.
—John Welwood[16]

Sadly, few of us get to stage 3. Our stage 2 disenchantment causes us to reject the other and mistrust relationships—or worse, our own heart. We may give up on our needs or plod ahead half-heartedly. What we don't realize is that while love is trustworthy, humans are conditional.[17] We love our partners when they are kind to us and fill our needs. We love them less, or not at all, when we find them challenging to be around, and especially when we perceive them as behaving uncharitably toward us. Then, we either move on or close our heart to love.

If we choose the naked path, we open up to our pain and disappointment. Rather than falling into despair, we appreciate the mysterious way that life—and this particular relationship—is growing us. What stops us from doing that right now? Most of us carry well into adulthood an infant-like wish for perfect attunement with another. We may not be able to put it consciously into words, but we often have a longing for continuous presence, praise, and positive mirroring.[18] An intimate relationship is supposed to be the place where such dreams really can come true. Romance culture not only perpetuates the wish for perfect togetherness well into adulthood but also propagates the myth of forever problem-free sex.

If our love story turns out to be more like the *Rocky Horror Picture Show*, which is how many of us experience disenchantment, it can be devastating. It is essential to feel the loss of our dream, or we may give up on love. We must grieve what we may not have had as a child and in likelihood what we will never have again—perfect attunement. Such an ending can be genuinely heartbreaking; we could describe it as the death of the dream person we have longed to love us.

The truth is, few of us know how to grieve. In our emotion-phobic culture, we've learned to take a pill or distract ourselves from painful emotions. However, grief serves an essential developmental purpose. When we allow old ideas, self-concepts, and limiting beliefs to die, and allow ourselves to grieve their passing, we open the possibility for an expanded, open, and curious consciousness. Grief isn't about resolution as is popularly understood, but about transformation, claims the psychotherapist and author Miriam Greenspan.[19]

Intimate partners will always grapple with irreconcilable differences. The gap between what your partner can provide and what you need to source from within is where spiritual practice flourishes. The perennial wisdom traditions tell us that the path to love—and freedom—involves resisting nothing. We create an opening for love and lifelong sexual engagement by accepting the "both/and" of life—which includes both joy and suffering. If we skirt the pain, we will eat enough to sustain ourselves without enjoying the deep nourishment of taking in all that life has to offer. The Lebanese American poet Kahlil Gibran writes:

> But, if in your fear you would seek only love's peace and love's
>     pleasure,
> Then it is better for you that you cover your nakedness
> and pass out of love's threshing-floor,
> Into the seasonless world where you shall laugh, but not
> all of your laughter, and weep, but not all of your tears.[20]

At stage 3, we consciously choose to take the naked path. If we successfully navigate this stage, we recognize that life—and by extension, love and sex—are full of problems and paradoxes. Moreover, nearly every growth spurt in life begins with some triggering event that throws the current order into chaos. Thus, the grief born of Cupid's leaden arrow offers an opportunity to shift how we relate to our habitual patterns, our partner, sex, and life as a whole.

## CRISIS OR OPPORTUNITY?

Beyond the ordinary trials and disappointments at stage 2, life sometimes throws us a devastating curveball, which only further disrupts the harmony of an erotic relationship.[21] While painful, without such "shock treatments," we might never wake up, claims Anaïs Nin.[22] The skills you can develop through awakened intimacy increase your chances of surviving these crises. They will help you meet these inevitable "pain points" with acceptance so that you can expand your pure erotic potential.

Here are five common pain points for stage 2 couples, although this is by no means an exhaustive list. We will experience a pain point before nearly every growth spurt in life. Sexually, have any of these five triggers affected you? If so, how have you expanded and contracted in response? Consider your reactions to the potential for growth these shock treatments provide.

**Sexual boredom** is often an invitation to become more fully alive. Perhaps a part of you has been whispering in your ear, and you haven't been listening carefully. It may be time to get out of those ruts that are stifling expression, verbally and sexually. However, boredom can also change by changing your attitude. If you believe the mystery is gone, you are likely to go on autopilot, thus perpetuating your ennui. Are you willing to cultivate a curious mind-set, even toward your boredom? Doing so can radically change how you experience your sex life.

An **outside attraction** can be fun or scary, possibly both. It dislodges the rock-solid feelings of "having" each other that can engender boredom in the first place. A sense of uncertainty can help you appreciate that being together is a choice, not a given. If boredom has led you to seek greener pastures, what would it take to reengage with your partner?

The **disclosure of an affair** can lead to a crisis and trigger deep feelings of betrayal. It can also be a catalyst for expansion. Many couples' therapists view the revelation of an affair as an opportunity to establish a new relationship contract. Depending on the circumstance, it might be possible to see an affair as marking the death of your old relationship, along with PEP-limiting patterns and beliefs. If so, can you participate in birthing a new one? When the dust settles, you may find that your bond is stronger than ever if you are honest about your needs and expectations.

Ruptures often occur because of **conflicting erotic preferences**. Each of us has a unique erotic palette, shaped in part by our early life. What happens when one of you wants to make an exotic dish part of the daily fare and the other has no taste for it? Such an impasse can also be a portal to connection and creativity if you work with your differences consciously and lovingly.

**Physical changes** can be harrowing, as they signal the loss of what we had believed was our unlimited vitality. Perhaps you are experiencing pain and reduced mobility due to illness or injury. As we will see in chapter 2, great sex has more to do with the state of our mind than with the function of our body. Nonetheless, age-related declines, such as erectile dysfunction (ED), are painful, especially if we equate sex with penetration.

While it may be worthwhile to explore an erectile enhancer, many sexual activities do not require a hard penis. Erectile dysfunction can be an opportunity to expand your repertoire, to focus not just on your genitals, but on your whole body as an erogenous zone. Likewise, menopause may require you to find a new rhythm, pace, and path to arousal than "business as usual."

As you can see, we will face numerous challenges individually, and as a couple. Our mind is the ultimate arbiter in determining whether an experience will make or break us, for how we interpret our experience determines how we respond to painful events. On the naked path, we recognize that many obstacles that appear to endanger our relationship can free us of deadening relational patterns. Leaning into these challenges instead of skirting these "pain points" is how we keep growing ourselves along with our pure erotic potential (see figure 1.1, "Maintain or Grow").

## YOUR PEP IS IN YOUR MIND: THE NOT-SO-SIMPLE ACT OF LETTING GO

We access our pure erotic potential by relinquishing goals, expectations, and inner models. In so doing, our lovemaking is fresh and

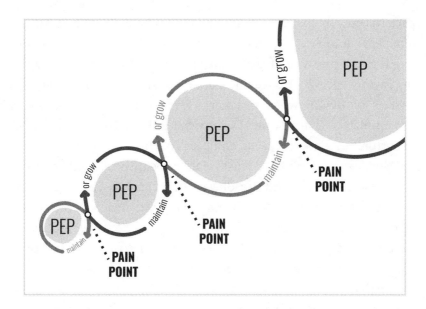

FIGURE 1.1 MAINTAIN OR GROW

A "pain point" precedes nearly every growth spurt. We can either address the issue mindfully and grow, or we can stay stuck at the barrier. Using your pain points for inner reflection can help your pure erotic potential flourish.

new every time. While "entering fresh" is the aspiration, in truth, we rarely meet eros, or life for that matter, in an unfiltered way. Our prior experiences shape our behaviors, feelings, and expectations automatically. That is, we enter each encounter expecting to be rewarded or disappointed, of hoping to experience pleasure or anticipating pain. Depending on our emotional and sexual history, these expectations will be pebbles or boulders on the road to our PEP.

At stage 1, our expectations temporarily loosen, and everything feels fresh and new. We often transcend our ordinary ways of relating and are open and exploratory, which heightens our feelings of enchantment. We may believe it is our behavior that is responsible for the resulting excitement, energy, and bliss we experience. However, this is mistaken; it is our open and exploratory *state of mind* that makes new sex exciting. Eventually, and inevitably, we will shrink away from this free state of pure erotic potential.

At stage 2, PEP-limiting mind-sets, imprints, and protective patterns only further eclipse this open field of possibility and greatly diminish our PEP. It is important that we examine these barriers. You might say, "I just want to get to the juicy part and have hot sex with my partner again." This feeling is understandable; however, like any "hero's journey" in which you search for something, face obstacles, and ultimately triumph over adversity, our PEP barriers turn out to be opportunities for personal and erotic expansion.

Most people don't know what is inhibiting their PEP until they do some research—not only by reading books and articles, but by looking inward. For instance, Abbey and Quinn honestly believed they were incompatible. They each felt the other was to blame for their problems. On the naked path, we consider barriers to be *internal* obstacles that are preventing us from being open, free, and spontaneous. It is for this reason that performance solutions may have little impact.

By taking the naked path, Abbey and Quinn discovered that the issues that were tearing them apart were not insurmountable and could become a bridge to wakeful erotic adventures. Now, six years into their relationship, they have a hopeful and realistic vision of their future together.

In my years working with couples, I have identified six common barriers on the path to realizing one's PEP (see figure 1.2, "PEP Barriers"). These barriers, or "checkpoints," are not sequential, nor are they necessarily a one-time pass. Individually, and as a couple, you may go through one or several on your journey. In each chapter, I will provide in-depth information on one or more barriers and show you the tools to work through them. Here are the six barriers and the chapters in which we discuss them; following the list is a brief discussion of each one.

1. Automaticity (chapters 1, 2, and 6)
2. Trances (chapters 1, 2, 5, and 6)
3. Fear of vulnerability and protective strategies (chapter 3)
4. The hidden factors (chapters 4 and 6)
5. Erotic wounds and trauma (chapter 4)
6. Shame (chapter 5)

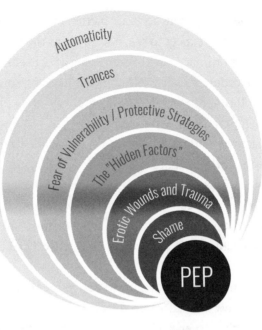

FIGURE 1.2 PEP BARRIERS

These barriers are like "checkpoints" on the naked path. You may have to work through one or more of these six inner obstacles to access your PEP.

## PEP-Barrier 1: Automaticity

Whether we are learning to walk or make love, automaticity follows us on the journey from novice to expert. Although the developmental feat of being able to tie your shoelaces automatically is a good thing, doing activities without paying attention inevitably leads to boredom. To regain our sense of erotic aliveness, we have to be present for sex.

Many PEP barriers are merely habits of body and mind, reinforced by automaticity. How many times have you mindlessly driven toward work when you were heading to the store? The same thing happens during sex. Our bodies will steer us where they have gone countless times before unless we are awake for the ride.

## PEP-Barrier 2: Trances

Until we wake up to it, we are all living in virtual reality. Mystics, Buddhist scholars, and researchers on consciousness assert that what we see and experience is not an accurate picture of reality. Our perceptual filters see what they expect to see, not things as they are.[23] Many go so far as to call our ordinary ways of perceiving a "consensual trance"[24] or the "trance of ordinary reality."[25] A trance is like a personal movie, with predictable plotlines in which our role is always the same, and others perform the functions we assign to them.

In my years of working with couples, I have identified three blockbuster movie plotlines that I see over and over again. In one movie, the doing side of sex seduces the protagonists. Like Ingrid and Walter mentioned above, we can become "sexual warriors," fighting our declining drive by trying new adventures. Such efforts are bound to the belief that we have to excel at sex to be worthy. I call this movie the performance trance.

In another movie, the protagonists resign themselves to deadening routines, somehow trapped in a production of *Groundhog Day* with a partner and sex life that never changes. I call this movie the familiarity trance.

In the third kind of movie, the protagonists believe their bond is fragile and that they must preserve it by hiding their fears, desires, and ultimately themselves. Like the trope of the secret operative, we may source aliveness covertly. Or, like Dorian Gray, we may resist change of any kind. I call this the safety trance.

These three trance states are poisons to our PEP—but we can learn to wake up from them.

## PEP-Barrier 3: Fear of Vulnerability and Protective Strategies

While mainstream culture tells us that we can live "happily ever after," growth occurs by rubbing up against each other rather than gliding over smooth ice. Stage 2 couples must wrestle with life's inevitable challenges. Many couples get stuck in impasses, terminate their relationship, or stop growing once they become disenchanted. Not understanding that intimacy elicits states of pain as well as pleasure, too many of us confuse conflict with incompatibility.

It may surprise you to hear that divisive sexual issues can bring you closer together. The key is to stay curious, truthful, and openhearted as you explore them. Unfortunately, most of us have learned to protect ourselves by hiding our vulnerability. We can transform challenging impasses into catalysts for connection by learning to share the hidden vulnerabilities at the core of our conflicts.

## PEP-Barrier 4: The Hidden Factors

We all receive messages about sex from our family and culture that dampen our erotic aliveness. Many of these messages encode before we are old enough to process them consciously. They are part of our early emotional learning. I call these imprints hidden factors because they are outside of awareness—until we make love.

Take a moment to think about this. Have you ever felt triggered when your partner touched you in a specific area? Have you felt sadness or fear during sex? You may have assumed these reactions are symptoms of your particular sexual dysfunction, but feeling triggered through sexual contact is common and natural.

In committed relationships, sex will eventually reveal these imprints like drift lines after high tide. When this happens, our efforts at renewed lovemaking can feel like jabbing at old wounds. If we are not aware of the potential for healing, in our response we may unconsciously find ourselves avoiding sex.

## PEP-Barrier 5: Erotic Wounds and Trauma

If you've been sexually wounded (a significant number of us have), you may experience shame because you can't "perform" like other people. You may view your limitations as impediments to sex and proof of your brokenness. The performance trance can also induce feelings of shame. We strive to conform to society's model of functional or "normal" sex instead of discovering and giving safe passage to our inside-out pathways to pleasure.

In truth, our PEP has nothing to do with functionality and everything to do with our consciousness. This view is the radicalness of *Passion and Presence*, and I hope a great relief to those of us who are unable to sustain erections or climax. As Maryann Camaroto reassures us: "We can sit next to our beloved index finger to index finger and have an orgasmic, heart-opening experience."[26] A mindful erotic portal can become a transformational path.

## PEP-Barrier 6: Shame

Many of us also assume that something is wrong with us when our arousal template differs from our model of what we think is normal or healthy sex. We may feel shame if our tastes are kinky, gender noncon-forming, or unlike our partner's preferences. Shame causes us to shut down or exile our erotic energy to the shadows. We are then more likely to hide or act out, which generates even more shame.

Naked sex involves more than taking off our clothes. We can es-tablish a couple's container in which it is safe to express our exiled or hidden impulses and desires. A couple that went to one of our retreats told me: "Our relationship feels like a whole new enterprise. Opening to my fantasies has taken loads of shame and guilt off my shoulders and has been fun and thrilling."

Many factors lead to erotic absence in long-term relationships. More-over, the inevitable encounter with our PEP barriers makes committed sex very naked. We can look at this phenomenon as bad and feel defeated and hopeless, or we can commit ourselves to awakened intimacy. On the naked path, we see and make use of the opportunity for growth and re-enchantment, even in the most challenging moments in our relationship. Such a path "gives us forward direction," says John Welwood.[27]

## MINDFUL ACTIVITIES AND NAKED REFLECTIONS

. . . . . . . . . . . . . . . . . . . . . . . . . . . . . . . . . . . . . . . . . . . . . . . . . . . . . . . . . . .

### Noticing Our Reactions to Having Goal-Free Sex

. . . . . . . . . . . . . . . . . . . . . . . . . . . . . . . . . . . . . . . . . . . . . . . . . . . . . . . . . . .

This exercise asks you to explore an imaginary sexual encounter that is without goals or comparisons.

Like a lot of people, you may want to get out of your sexual rut and feel free again but might also feel afraid of being too much, not doing it right, feeling exposed, or being judged. These fears are shared by many, in fact, are almost universal. You might begin to realize how they also diminish your PEP. In this exercise, we can safely explore our PEP and share what emerges through the lens of no judgment.

If you are doing this exercise with a partner, make sure each of you completes the activity separately before sharing your observations.

## Part 1: Prepare

Start by closing your eyes and taking several deep breaths. Then, allow yourself to imagine you have not seen sex on television, or anywhere, and you have not had sex with your partner.

## Part 2: Explore

From this "blank slate" mind-set, imagine a sexual encounter with your partner where there is no past to compare to, no goal to achieve. You are merely listening inside, feeling yourself, and giving your unshaped, unscripted impulses free expression.

Let images surface and impulses roam without the confines of what has happened in previous encounters. Continue to imagine opening to what is unfolding here and now, instead of taking familiar paths to arousal.

## Part 3: Observe

Begin to notice what parts of you come alive in this experience. What feelings and emotions emerge as you try on this boundless erotic potential?

Take your time as you study the range of your responses, including images, feelings, and physical sensations.

Notice anything that stops you or wants to limit self-expression—perhaps a voice, an image, a memory, or some fear or embarrassment. Take your time as you explore this. Be curious.

## Naked Reflections

If possible, and desired, share what emerged from the exercise with your partner.

What aspects of your experience were surprising to you? What opens up in you with the possibility of goal-free sex? What seems to want to close you down?

Take a moment also to share how it is to speak with each other about this.

# 2.

# EROTIC PRESENCE

## Cultivating a State of Mind for Intimate and Creative Sex

Two years after sending their introductory email, signed "Desperate in Dorchester," Carla and Miguel are finally able to attend one of my couples' Passion and Presence retreats. As I listen to Carla describe the adventures she and Miguel had at the beginning of their relationship, I can feel her longing to get back there. That period of heightened arousal is, evidently, Carla's only reference for exciting and fulfilling sex. When I explain that she was having sex on steroids back then, Carla laughs, and Miguel wonders if Carla can refill her prescription. However, their mood sours when they describe their current sex life.

As parents of three children with special needs, the couple has spent a decade meeting with a variety of specialists instead of lingering in bed. Both have demanding jobs: Miguel works as an ER nurse in the evenings, and Carla is an account manager at a large public relations firm. As is often the case for busy stage 2 couples, making time for sex has fallen to the bottom of their to-do lists—their occasional hook-ups are likely to happen at 5:45 in the morning.

Miguel gives me a rundown of these encounters, and I can see why they are wistful. While Carla prefers to build up to genital contact, with no time to spare before their kids wake up, she usually lets him bring her to orgasm through oral sex. Then, Miguel enters Carla for a minute

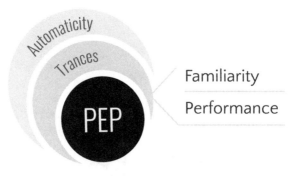

FIGURE 2.1 CHAPTER 2 PEP BARRIERS

or two to finish himself off. Although this scenario "works" it is hardly inspiring, especially to Carla, whose fantasy life features seduction and danger. Miguel also admits that he longs to feel more connected to Carla when they make love.

Relying on a "tried and true" path to orgasm stifles eros. Moreover, this couple's routine is marginally satisfying, physically, but leaves them hungry in every other way. Carla and Miguel are mesmerized by the familiarity trance, and miles away from their PEP.

## WAKE ME WHEN IT'S OVER: THE FAMILIARITY TRANCE

Few—if any—of us escape the familiarity trance. We expect what we call sexual boredom to be inevitable, if not something permanent once it has set in. Despite this, we still yearn for stage 1, when our every sexual encounter was an excursion to somewhere new, an unscripted meeting of two open and curious beings.

By the time our sexual intensity fizzles at stage 2, it is merely a matter of time before automaticity comes to replace our spirit of adventure. If exhaustion accompanies our disenchantment, we will find ourselves sleepwalking through sex, repeating the same moves over and over.

*Automaticity is the first and perhaps most substantial barrier to our PEP.* However, in many instances, sexual boredom is nothing more than succumbing to numbing habits and routines, as we've seen with Carla and

Miguel. At stage 2, we've memorized each other's erogenous zones, and now because of a shortage of time and limiting mind-sets, we automatically take shortcuts to arousal. We lose our "anything is possible" state of mind and go for the sure bet every time. Unfortunately, by avoiding the hazards (and delights!) of curiosity and uncertainty, we close the doors to our PEP. Cultivating erotic presence is how we open them again.

## Trance-Induced Blindness

The absence of satisfying sex at stage 2 can take the joy out of living. Many couples disengage sexually, often leading one or both partners to source aliveness elsewhere. Six months before I met with Carla and Miguel, Carla began an affair with a woman who worked in the art department at her company. The two spent long hours together producing collateral material for an important campaign. Once their after-hours conversations moved from the project to their personal lives, Carla found herself on the receiving end of Porsha's undivided attention.

This attention was exhilarating; it rekindled something of the feelings of enchantment she experienced with Miguel those many years ago. For when Carla and Miguel first got together, they talked endlessly about everything and listened to each other with rapt attention. Now, after sixteen years of marriage, they only half-listen when the other speaks, rarely sitting down together except to talk about their children.

While the phrase "I only have eyes for you" is a powerful aphrodisiac for enchanted stage 1 couples, this tunnel vision is always short-lived. Human brains (and loins) light up for novelty. We learn and also survive by paying attention to new things. However, once we become familiar with something, we see what we expect to see instead of what's there.[1]

Neuroscientists tell us that our habits of perception determine what we pay attention to *and* what we ignore.[2] When we are enchanted, we disregard anything that doesn't fit our inflated vision of our beloved. Unfortunately, the blinders of the familiarity trance are equally cursed. At stage 2, we fail to register behaviors in our partner that are surprising and new simply because we stop looking for them.

Trance-induced blindness explains why so many people fail the "Notice anything different about me?" test and why that failure is so crushing. The resulting blow has little to do with a new haircut, but rather a deeper wound about not being seen anymore. The familiar person is our emotional anchor but also becomes someone we can take for granted. Eventually, and inevitably, trance-induced blindness leads to trance-induced boredom.

While our feelings of boredom are real, they usually have little to do with the person who bores us. We might even think we know everything there is to know about our partner, but research points to the contrary. In one study, couples that had been together for less than two years predicted their partner's preferences better than those that had been together much longer.[3] Nonetheless, our false sense of knowing all there is diminishes our curiosity and presence[4]—and therefore our PEP.

## Removing Our Blinders

Carla and Miguel took the affair as a wake-up call. They tell me they are eager to reinvigorate their erotic life but haven't a clue where to start. I explain that Cupid's leaden arrow has sent them into a deep sleep. So how can they use Cupid's wings to make magic from the ordinary? I recommend they do an activity called "Seeing Fresh" (see the end of this chapter) regularly to help them enlarge their perceptual filters. Recognizing that we have been conditioned to see things a certain way is an essential aspect of awakened intimacy.

How we perceive our partners and react during sex are the products of our internal organizers of experience, most of which are unconscious. They filter what we see and experience in accord with our beliefs and expectations.[5] Just as we wake from a dream into a larger reality, our normal states of existence are only a small slice of what might be outside of our myopic view. Until we wake up to the possibility of a broader perspective, we could go as far as to say that our view of our relationship is embedded in trance states.

When we are in the familiarity trance, we refrain from trying new things because we "know" our partner won't be receptive to them. We miss signals of responsiveness because we point our attention elsewhere. Having decided the mystery is gone, we go through the motions or switch on a fantasy. Like Carla, we may start to wonder what it would be like to have sex with other people.

Pitching a curiosity for the great unknown against the predictability of life with a partner of some years is natural. It expresses our inborn longing to learn through new experiences. When viewed this way, feelings of restlessness can signal the readiness to grow beyond routine and maintenance to fulfill our evolutionary potential to transform. So, how can we become reenchanted with each other again?

When we find our sex life to be unsatisfactory, we often look outside ourselves for the answer. We may source variety from novel positions, apparel, and toys (the "novelty trap") rather than discovering something new *between* us. We don't realize that our beliefs and expectations are the cause of our suffering. Such a misconception of reality is called "ignorance" in Buddhism. The antidote for this "poison" is to see things as they are.[6]

## THE POWER OF PRESENCE: OVERCOMING AUTOMATICITY

To recover a sense of erotic mystery, I encourage Carla and Miguel to go "off script." I instruct them to *stop and start over* whenever they are slipping into their routine and to let go of the goal of having an orgasm. When we practice erotic presence, we can stop and start over each time we default to a numbing routine. Otherwise, our automated programs in all likelihood will continue to run our lives.

My next suggestion amuses them: "If something feels good, don't repeat it the next time!" This advice goes against popular thinking. We're taught to find something that works and to stick with it. But herein lies the problem: Mindless repetition becomes habit-driven sex. We may experience release, but not the deep satisfaction that comes from taking a new turn. It is through the cultivation of erotic presence that we see fresh and access the creativity at the core of our PEP.

Carla and Miguel start on their naked path as soon as they agree to take themselves off their well-trodden sexual path. As they cultivate erotic presence, they begin to wake up from the hypnotic effect of their

PEP-limiting trances and automaticity. We will see how things turn out for the "desperate" couple when we meet them again in chapter 5.

## BIGGER, BETTER, MORE: THE PERFORMANCE TRANCE

As sexual intensity wanes with familiarity, some couples go to Herculean efforts to restore their flagging drive—recall Walter and Ingrid. Walter, a high-powered New York attorney, was seduced by the culture of perfectionism.[7] This translated at home into the performance trance: he and Ingrid had been trying to resolve their sexual problems by learning new techniques, such as Tantra and light bondage.

Great sex is a mind-set, not a skill set. The performance trance is fused with the "Olympian imperative" to excel at everything we do, including sex. When we operate within the performance model, not only do we become less attuned to what's happening inside of us, but we also lose contact with our innate eroticism. In fact, our focus is on being "hot," pleasing our partner, and doing it "right" instead of what we are feeling. When Walter and Ingrid take in these ideas, Ingrid's face softens, and Walter sits back in his chair.

Looking for a way to drive this point home more and knowing that Walter and Ingrid have two teenage daughters, I mention the book *Girls and Sex*, in which Peggy Orenstein writes that a whole new generation of girls are more concerned with how their body looks to someone else than how it feels to them.[8] They exchange glances. This outside-in orientation increases anxiety for *all* of us. I turn to Walter who I know worries about erectile dysfunction. "If we couple sex with competency, or penetration, we may avoid physical contact because we don't want to 'start something we can't finish.'" He nods.

The "bigger, better, more" mentality that pervades the performance trance is PEP-inhibiting. Our efforts to have more or better sex often lead us to feel unfulfilled and insecure. In Buddhism, this quality of grasping for more is called "greed."[9] It can also be accompanied by a hell-bent determination to "succeed" despite the consequences for ourselves and others. In the case of sex, we mistakenly think wherever we are heading is where the pleasure lies, but we are pointed in the wrong direction.

PEP has nothing to do with techniques, prowess, or performance. It depends on one thing only—your state of mind. The good news is that passion and novelty can still be yours. Instead of scouring the sexual marketplace for new thrills, I suggest that Walter and Ingrid work with their minds to find novelty. I explain that our state of mind determines the quality of our sex life much more than what we *do* in bed. They are skeptical but curious.

If you are skeptical too, try this thought experiment: take one minute for each scenario to notice anything that changes in your experience when you imagine having sex with only this sole purpose in mind:

### Scenario #1: Having sex for physical release

(*What do you imagine is happening during the encounter? How does your body feel? What is your relationship with your partner? Which parts of you are engaging? Which parts of you are stepping back?*)

### Scenario #2: Having sex to merge with the "great all" (i.e., mystery, the divine, nature, however this resonates for you)

(*What do you imagine is happening during the encounter? How does your body feel? What is your relationship with your partner? Which parts of you are engaging? Which parts of you are stepping back?*)

### Scenario #3: Having sex to feel close and connected

(*What do you imagine is happening during the encounter? How does your body feel? What is your relationship with your partner? Which parts of you are engaging? Which parts of you are stepping back?*)

Did you sense something change in your attitude, energy, and physical response to these different scenarios? If so, those changes began in your head, not in your bed. Our state of mind determines how we show up for sex and what we experience when we have it. It is common to harbor PEP-limiting mind-sets. These mind-sets tell us there is nothing new here or that we have to power through sex to reach a goal. Mindfulness and erotic presence can help us recover together the mystery, creativity, and depth of connection that diminish over time.

Now let's bring this idea home, literally.

**Scenario #4: Take a moment to consider having sex with your partner as you usually have it. Make this mental exercise as real as possible. What do you anticipate will happen? Run it through like a "little movie."**

*(How does your body feel? What is your relationship with your partner? Which parts of you are engaging? Which parts of you are stepping back?)*

Pause to notice how your expectations are shaping your attitude and physical responses right now. If you are feeling anything but excitement, try to cultivate a state of mind attuned to novelty, as if it is the first time you will be together. Don't rely on going back in time to a stage 1 memory; let your imagination be awake to the here and now with your partner. Just by entering a sexual encounter as if it is the first and only time together generates thrill and uncertainty and also wakes up your PEP.

The gifts of working with our minds extend far beyond having better sex. Awakening from automaticity enables us to engage more fully with life. We loosen limiting habits of all kinds, which leads us to greater wisdom and freedom.[10] In this way, our sexual relationship can support growth on many levels and become a transformational path. Stage 3 couples capitalize on this growth-inducing opportunity and so can you. They cultivate qualities of mind that increase pleasure and awareness by staying present during sex.

## OVERCOMING PEP-LIMITING MIND-SETS WITH MINDFULNESS

Once considered a fringe activity known mostly to Buddhists, mindfulness has gone mainstream.[11] Media celebrities such as Anderson Cooper and Dan Harris have espoused mindfulness as a near-panacea for stress, pain reduction, and workplace productivity.[12] This enthusiasm is not all hype, either. A hoard of research extols the physical, emotional, and mental benefits of regular mindfulness practice,[13] many of which transfer to sex. What's more, mindfulness is not just a New Age practice or passing fancy. Eighteen million people meditate according to a survey by the National Institute of Health, and by several indicators, that number is climbing.[14]

Why does following our breath in a nonjudging way (the most common mindfulness practice) have such widespread appeal? Is it because becoming mindful defies the "fast and furious" pace that drives most people's lives? The swelling mindfulness movement seems to suggest a cultural shift from doing to being, from accomplishing to savoring, and from acting automatically to becoming conscious of the subtle inner processes that lead us to act (or act out) in habitual ways.

While today mindfulness is often used to manage stress and enhance productivity, the original intent of this 2,500-year-old practice was to become awakened,[15] which means present and fully aware rather than fixated or automatic. It also means being in the fullness of life rather than in a trance.[16] Trance-induced blindness can prevent us from seeing that our partner has new and different desires than when we first met them one or ten years ago. We can never awaken our intimacy unless we wake up to any fixed ideas we are holding about our partner, ourselves, and sex.

However, when we are in a trance, we take our narrow and distorted view of reality as truth.[17] In such moments, we become identified with our feelings and perceptions, just as we might mistake panic-induced palpitations for a heart attack. Even though the danger is not life-threatening, our world shrinks to a fight for survival. The therapist and writer Steven Stosney explains, "If there's no obvious exception to the string of assumptions underlying a given behavioral impulse, we act without conscious thought, emotion or perception of action."[18] In other words, we are entirely automatic.

In Eastern traditions, we escape the pull of automaticity by cultivating an "internal observer." In truth, the observer is more a quality of awareness that we can develop through meditation rather than a separate part of ourselves. This internal observer helps us notice our habits of mind in real time. When something we do becomes a habit, it is likely unconscious. Therefore, when we meditate it can be a shock to observe our patterns dancing in front of our eyes.

We may be surprised to discover that we are judging others and ourselves much of the time. Alternatively, we may notice how we are constantly worrying about things that haven't happened yet or have already happened. We may see our habit of leaving our experience instead of lingering with the raw intensity of our anguish or grief. In fact, as anyone who meditates knows, we are absent a great deal of the time.

We can cultivate this awareness of being present if we practice mindfulness regularly. Every time we notice we have traveled to a judgment or projection we can come back to the present moment. Every time our world shrinks from an open state of flow to a faultfinding loop, we can unhook by coming back to the fullness of the moment. Mindfulness is our remedy for absence and our automaticity in bed. We can use mindfulness to overcome PEP-limiting mind-sets and trance states that diminish our erotic creativity and create dissatisfaction in our long-term relationship.

As Tara Healey at Harvard Pilgrim Health Care puts it, "Mindfulness interrupts the conditioned responses that prevent us from exploring new avenues of thought, choking our creative potential."[19] Standing up "against a habit," as she says, weakens the "grip of our conditioning." Although we might be familiar with how to apply mindfulness in our work setting, I call mindfulness, in the context of sex, erotic presence. Without it, our body might be there, but our mind is not.

I hope by now you are seeing that we do not need to buy a prop or enact a role-play to reengage our curiosity, nor do we need to continue to rely on predictable routines. When curiosity ebbs at stage 2, practicing erotic presence can restore it. When we are present with each other, we can key off of the energy unfolding between us. We begin to notice many pathways to pleasure that are available in the here and now and to follow them—not because we are focused on the destination, but because we are here for the ride. Cultivating erotic presence can revitalize your sex life and help you access your PEP.

Unfortunately, as we've seen, it is hard to stay present to familiar things. The first time we do anything we are very attentive, but soon after, automaticity takes over. How often do we look without seeing? Hear without listening? Eat without tasting? Absence may make the heart grow fonder when we are miles away geographically, but our absence in the bedroom only diminishes our PEP.

It's paradoxical, but we become present as soon as we notice our absence. Whenever we get swept up in thoughts or lulled into the familiarity trance, we can gently bring awareness back to the moment. This mindful approach is the essence of the perennial wisdom traditions and essential to the naked path.

## TAKING IT TO THE SHEETS: MINDFUL SEX

So, what exactly is mindful sex? What images come into your mind at the mention of "erotic presence"? Are you seeing two people breathing in synchrony as they gaze lovingly into each other's eyes? If you imagine penetration, are you seeing slow thrusts?

Mindful sex is not necessarily "slow sex." Nor is it an alternative to lusty or even "rough" sex. Any kind of sex can be mindful. It is the quality of presence that we bring to whatever type of sex we are having right now. This presence is curious and allowing. With erotic presence, we can feel ourselves emotionally, energetically, and physically. The inner observer has open eyes, enabling us to notice our thoughts, habits, and impulses throughout the experience.

Although there is no single experience of mindful sex, I've identified five features that make it a wakeful adventure. Some of these features reflect the spirit or attitude of mindful sex; others refer to the practice or state of consciousness that supports being open and wakeful.

*The Five Features of Mindful Sex*
1. Eliminating goals and reference points
2. Embracing both the joys and challenges bundled with sex
3. Accepting the impermanence that runs through our erotic life
4. Cultivating a state of novelty
5. Becoming present and embodied

Let's look at the list in more depth. Each of the five features begins with a question or set of questions.

## 1. Eliminating Goals and Reference Points

*How would it be to enter an erotic experience without a destination or frame of reference?*

Mindful sex keeps us coming back to the "spacious mind" of our pure erotic potential. In this state, we are free from goals and reference points that stifle the potential creativity available in the here and now. We practice noticing—again and again—when we are becoming automatic or goal oriented. At such times, we pause and wait for the next impulse to see where it might take us rather than plowing ahead.

From a spacious mind, we might find ourselves drawn to stroking our partner's body in a new way. Alternatively, we may become newly aware of where and how we want to be touched at this moment. When we release ourselves from "destination tyranny" by emptying our mind of goals and reference points, we become curious explorers. We accept like any intrepid adventurer that sometimes the path we thought was to an exotic mushroom turns out to be a muddy dead end. With a spacious mind, we *re-wild* our sex life by exploring new trails.

## 2. Embracing Both the Joys and Challenges Bundled with Sex

*Do you assume that sex should always be good, if not great?*

When it comes to sex, most of us chase pleasure and judge challenges and "just okay" sex as bad news. However, real-life sex can have incredible highs as well as multiple frustrations, just as real-life vacations can include flight delays or bungled hotel reservations. While we may believe that sex should be consistently fulfilling, many sexual experiences are okay, at best. Research tells us that more than 50 percent of the time, sex will be more enjoyable for one of us than the other.[20]

Expecting sex always to be comfortable and satisfying is like hoping the weather will be sunny 365 days of the year. Like the weather, our sex life can be hot and steamy, stormy, or dry. We can be in a drought for months, even years. Nevertheless, couples who claim togetherness in sickness and health may lose said devotion when their sex life goes south. With mindfulness, we can begin to embrace the full range of our sexual experiences as a couple as we develop a nonjudgmental attitude toward them all.

Stage 3 couples do just that; they appreciate their delightful, deeply satisfying encounters as well as those that are awkward and disappointing. They shift their orientation so that sexual variability is merely evidence of the mystery of eros, rather than a problem to solve. With this mind-set, even unsatisfying experiences become grist for the mill. As Sengstan put it in the *Hsin Hsin Ming*, "The Great Way is not difficult for those who have no preferences."[21]

## 3. Accepting the Impermanence That Runs through Our Erotic Life

*Are you willing to surrender your attachment to a particular outcome or view of "great sex"? Can you let go of the so-called good times and bad?*

Why do intense moments of pleasure only slip through our grasp when we try to recapture them later? Our best sexual experiences are like soap bubbles, delicate and short-lived. Even the Big O is normally only seven to twenty seconds long. Trying to keep our sex life the same is like saving a pressed flower. It will forever be just an echo of its former self, lifeless and without fragrance.

The good news is that something as good or better than your best sex is waiting for you right now. You will miss it if you try to reprise the oldies but goodies, or judge your sex life by your last few unsatisfying encounters. As you may have seen in the thought experiment earlier, our expectations determine what is possible between us. If we have the idea that our sex life is a problem, we are likely to be cautious and avoidant of sex.

Mindfulness can help us not attach to a particular experience of sex—good or bad. It can release every sexual experience back into the stream of ongoing experiences we are likely to have as a couple. Having goals can create attachment toward future experiences and cause rejection of current moments together. Holding on to reference points can lead us to want to replicate past experiences, the satisfying as well as the unsatisfying. When we let go of our attachment to specific experiences, we allow ourselves to discover pathways to pleasure that fit what is realistic and desirable for us right now.

If your sex life has been less than wonderful, try to empty yourself of expectations and inner models. This practice is what stage 3 couples do each time they make love. They release their images of what their best and worst sex is like and meet freshly. If you let go of your reference points, then whatever is happening right now *is* your "best sex."

## 4. Cultivating a State of Novelty

*In a spirit of exploration, are you willing to see how mindfulness can convert an ordinary and familiar sexual encounter into something novel?*

Ellen Langer is a social psychologist at Harvard University who has been studying mindfulness for more than forty years. Her findings indicate that when we look for novelty in familiar places, we anchor ourselves in the present.[22] Because we are engaged, we enjoy ourselves and are more creative. I believe she's right.

Mindful sex follows an internal rhythm, not a sexual script. We listen inside for the eros energy that pulses through us. When we liberate ourselves from the pressure to reach a goal and erase our images of sex, our experience becomes a free-form jam session. Instead of kissing our partner's body with our lips, we might draw different shapes with our tongue, making a painting with our mouth. Instead of going up and down with our head, we might zigzag across our partner's genitals and hum, enjoying the vibrations we feel inside of our mouth.

We awaken our PEP by following erotic impulses as they arise moment to moment without succumbing to automatic moves and routines. Sometimes our riffs will be mind-blowing, sometimes one or both of us may not be feeling the music. Whatever happens is okay. Acceptance is a crucial element of traditional mindfulness as well as mindful sex.

By improvising instead of playing tired standards, we access infinite possibilities rather than going straight for an orgasm. Of course, not every single stroke, kiss, or lick will be a first. However, the combination will be unique, and so will the energy behind it. Our playfulness,

passion, and intimacy are born of the moment and therefore are fresh
and unrepeatable.

## 5. Becoming Present and Embodied

*What if you want to feel aroused but have trouble doing so? How does
sensation get coded as pleasure?*

Some of us have bodies that talk to us through a megaphone. Our
internal sensations may be so intense that we want to cover our ears.
Others of us can go all day long without eating or drinking and never
feeling hunger or thirst. Mindfulness can help you feel yourself from the
inside, including your turn-on. This process is called "interoception."
When you link your pounding chest to fear and your growling stomach
to hunger, you are using interoception, or your "felt sense."[23] The same
system helps you recognize sexual arousal.[24]

The brain's insula is ground control for your felt sense. It is the re-
lay station between body and brain and supports erotic attunement.[25]
Research by Sara Lazar indicates that mindfulness practice thickens
the insula.[26] In one study, this resulted in more intense orgasms for
women.[27] British Columbia's Sexual Health Lab provides conclusive
evidence that mindfulness can restore desire, arousal, and sexual functioning in women with arousal disorders related to gynecological cancer and sexual abuse.[28]

Developing your sexual felt sense is essential to erotic attunement,
which is the ability to feel your partner while you are feeling yourself
during an erotic exchange. As we will see in chapter 6, the art of mindful
sex is learning how to engage in an unscripted call-and-response. We do
this by feeling and responding to each other's nonverbal cues.

You can develop your sexual felt sense by telescoping in on the sensations in your body that accompany arousal. When you bring focused
attention to the body, you converse with your nervous system. Corre-
sponding regions of your brain light up in the places where you are receiving physical contact, but only if you bring awareness to those areas.[29]

If you are receiving *wanted* sexual stimulation, your feelings of
arousal and your genital response synch up, resulting in "sexual concordance." The higher your brain-genital concordance, the more likely

you are to experience pleasure during sex.[30] You can increase this concordance by using mindful awareness to notice the *feel of the feelings* you experience when you touch yourself and when your partner licks, kisses, sucks, or scratches you in different parts of your body.[31]

Focused awareness on the body counters our tendency to go into our head and builds our capacity to concentrate and stay present. Each time your mind goes anywhere but here, gently bring it back to the body via your senses. If you are distracted or numb, you won't notice the richness of the moment, and you won't experience the pleasure-enhancing benefits of sexual concordance. By becoming present and embodied, you can experience new worlds without leaving the bedroom.

## BEYOND THE BODY: WAKEFUL SEX

Sensing at the body level builds concentration and enhances sexual concordance. We can also go wide-angle. We can use the "open focus" of our awareness to notice how our life themes, limiting beliefs, and habitual behaviors display themselves on the erotic stage. By seeing, and then pausing and studying our experience moment by moment, we bring awareness to the customarily hidden shapers of our experience. "Wakeful sex" wakes us up from our habits and trances.

We may start to ask newer questions of ourselves. For example: Are we waiting for our partner to initiate because we feel too shy to do so ourselves? We may wonder how giving up on shaping an erotic experience expresses our relationship to power. Does hiding our sexual wishes protect us from disappointment or reflect an underlying belief that other people's needs are more important than our own? What do our habits regarding initiating, expressing, giving, and receiving tell us about our early conditioning? What did we imprint about sex? About pleasure? About love?

We can investigate everything that diminishes our PEP, including protective strategies and the emotions behind them. For example, with the help of mindful awareness, we recognize that after sex, we are chronically dissatisfied. By staying curious, we notice that underneath our dissatisfaction is an unwillingness to ask for what we want. Beneath our reluctance is the fear that something is wrong with us for having "kinky" desires in the first place. And, behind that is our shame. Voilà!

## WAKING UP, GENTLY

The things we can notice when we have sex mindfully are endless. However, as our PEP-limiting tendencies become visible to us, we may fear that our habits are too entrenched for us to experience anything new with our long-term partner. We may believe we have too many internal roadblocks to ever come close to our PEP. In turn, we may judge ourselves or want to give up the practice of mindful sex.

It is natural to become discouraged when we see the usually hidden aspects of our mental and emotional life. It is for this reason that meditation teachers throughout the ages have encouraged practitioners to stay loving and curious toward themselves as they observe their habitual patterns. Self-aggression is the wrong spirit. Waking up is an act of love, not a whack on the head. "It is only when we begin to relax with ourselves as we are that meditation becomes a transformative process," claims the American Tibetan nun and author Pema Chödrön.[32]

Waking ourselves up is a lifelong project, not a race. Falling into a trance state is not unique to sex; we will fall into trance states whenever we fall asleep, even briefly. Many things, including automatic scrolling on our phones, can create a trancelike state. Our tendency to sleepwalk through life—and especially sex—is why regular mindfulness practice is essential. New habits are hard-won but can take hold with training, intention, and willingness to face the "pull" of our old ways.

In Sanskrit, the word *mukta* means "released." The intent of mindfulness within Buddhism was to help us to recognize and find relief from suffering born of a misapprehension of reality. Mindfulness helps us gently wake up from distorted perceptions and beliefs that have become automatized and can lead to trancelike states. We can learn to shift from being fused with such states to becoming a curious and compassionate witness to our states.[33]

This process is called "disidentification" (see figure 2.2, "Disidentification"). Disidentification is like going into a bigger room. Instead of

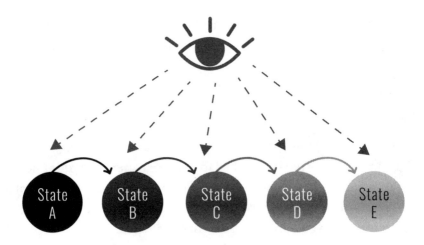

**FIGURE 2.2 DISIDENTIFICATION**

—from Halko Weiss

When we are in a trance, we view reality from inside the circle of our state. The "internal observer" gives us the sky view so we can wake up from our myopic view.

seeing just the bedroom, we see the entire house. Instead of seeing only the house, we see the whole neighborhood. And, with each widening of perception, we become wiser, have more choices, and access more PEP. A regular mindfulness practice can help us cultivate the inner observer as we free ourselves from trance states and PEP-limiting mind-sets.

## Waking Up from the Performance Trance

Are you ready to let go of a "bigger, better, more" mentality?

Sex sells. Advertisers, movie producers, and book publishers capitalize on this fact. Unfortunately, the media's portrayal of eroticism perpetuates a myth that partner sex is always hot, mutually satisfying, and spontaneous. It isn't, but you already know this. Or do you?

Enticed by the enjoinder to "be the best we can be," many of us go to great lengths to become sexual Olympians—learning techniques to become masterful lovers instead of discovering inside-out pathways to pleasure. The naked truth is this: satisfaction lies in the call-and-response of two attuned people who are not aiming but are letting eros lead.

In performance trance, we forget this. We strive to reach specific benchmarks like arousal, orgasm, or intercourse. Our attention turns away from the moment to concerns about competency: We silently wonder, am I wet, hard, or sexy enough? Is my technique okay? Usually, we answer ourselves with a "no." The danger of this trance is that we will never be a "good-enough" lover, and this can only mean, in all likelihood, that we will never have "good-enough" sex.

Mindfulness is an antidote to the "bigger, better, more" mentality that undergirds the performance trance. As we saw in the first of the five features listed above, we release ourselves from destination tyranny when we pause and savor the moment. If we notice we are striving for the next great thing, we pause to regain a spirit of exploration that is guided by our curiosity. As we shift from performing to exploring, we realize that our PEP has nothing to do with being an accomplished lover. An achievement mentality only creates sexual anxiety and leads to avoidance, warns the researchers Barry McCarthy and Lana Wald.[34]

Remember Walter and Ingrid? Four months after our first meeting, the couple returned for part 2 of our Tending Eros series. The tension I felt being with them before had all but disappeared, along with the toe-tapping restlessness I had noted in Walter. I'm eager to hear about their journey, but avoid steering the session with too firm a hand. I wait, and surprisingly, so do they.

We look at each other for about a minute; then Walter begins: "I'll be honest, it took some time for us to surrender our 'fight mode,' as you called it. I've been competitive all my life. Everything I have has come from my effort and determination." He continues by saying, "I'm a pragmatist, and if my strategy isn't getting me results, I'm willing to try a different approach. One day on the train, I read something that reminded me of what you said at the last retreat about the cult of perfection and the 'Olympian imperative' to score a perfect 10 in all areas of life."[35]

Walter continues, "A few days after we got back, we agreed that every single time I was straining to make something happen during sex, we would stop." Ingrid laughs, "That was about ten times in the first two minutes." She continues, "Sex had always been a serious business for us, but we just kept laughing. It got so ridiculous that we thought we would never get to sex, but at one point we just looked into each other's eyes and something shifted." *They are looking at each other that way right now. It is intimate and loving.* "Walter held me, and his eyes welled up," says Ingrid, speaking more softly than moments before. "I could feel he was in his heart." Again, they pause to look at each other.

"We decided to play the impulse game you told us about in the retreat. Walter asked, 'What's your impulse?' Surprisingly, I wanted to be tied up."

If we are present and listening inside, we may want to add a prop or toy, which is different from artificially incorporating something into our lovemaking to fill the novelty prescription.

Ingrid continues, "Walter went into the garage to get some rope, but it didn't feel right. I suggested he grab the silk belt off my robe. Then, I asked him, 'What's *your* impulse?' and he said, 'To tie your wrists to the bedposts.' We were still playful, but I also felt nervous. I am usually very active during sex. In fact, until that moment, I hadn't realized how much control I like to have during sex. I paused to study my reaction, and we talked about it, which was also new. I like to use my hands to stimulate Walter, but I couldn't. We remembered you telling us to let whatever is coming up be part of the dance. So, we tried to think of a way that I could be passive *and* in control."

"Here's where it gets fun," says Walter. "We decided that Ingrid would tell me what to do. If I did what she asked, she would stroke me with her feet. If I didn't do it exactly right, she would use her feet to push me away." "It was exciting and awkward because I couldn't use my hands to stimulate Walter like I usually do," Ingrid adds. "Nothing we were doing felt natural. That's when I realized how goal oriented *I* am. It's not just Walter."

Self-awareness is the gift of mindful sex. We notice our tendencies by observing how we are feeling and behaving while making love. Instead of avoiding unpleasant feelings, we pause to study them. We choose to make necessary adjustments to feel more comfortable and use our discoveries to shift habits that may no longer be serving us.

Ingrid continues, "I decided that instead of trying to pleasure Walter, that I would taste and smell him. Surprisingly, I could feel more of myself when I did that. I noticed small waves of arousal moved through my body when Walter put his penis inside my mouth. I thought of the image of the homunculus you showed us at the retreat with those big swollen lips, and I decided to feel the nerve endings inside of my lips. I just kept staying curious and open, feeling the different sensations in my mouth."

"Eventually, my arms got tired, so I asked Walter to untie me." Walter decides now is a good time to chime in. "I really wanted to be inside of Ingrid and was starting to mount her in my usual missionary way, but instead, we decided to lie on our sides and face each other." "That was almost too much," Ingrid admits, but I can see that Walter is looking at Ingrid with admiration. They continue telling me more details of their sex play, including the moment when they paused because they were losing aliveness. Ingrid explains, "I needed to know that Walter was okay with all this, and he told me that he was." "It sounds like you believed him," I say. She searches his face now for confirmation and Walter nods.

"That evening was unique, for sure," says Walter. "We haven't had anything quite like that adventure since, but it hasn't been 'business as usual' either." I reiterate that sex can be a creative improvisation when we surrender goals and are present to the moment. This potential doesn't mean that every experience will be fantastic, but that is okay.

Inevitably, we will sometimes fall back on our patterns, especially when we are tired, because presence is expensive, energy-wise.[36] Automaticity enables us to do things *without* having a presence of mind. However, Ingrid and Walter now know that the possibilities are endless when they listen inside for the next impulse instead of pushing to reach a goal. They can relax during sex and make things up as they go along. They realize that how they *are* during sex shapes their experience much more than what they do in bed.

## Waking Up from the Familiarity Trance by Recovering Curiosity Again and Again

In the familiarity trance, we approach sex with the same tired eyes. We let our bodies do what they do without being awake to the experience unfolding between us. Mindfulness trains us to meet fresh every time. Instead of fixing our partner to the first frame of a lifelong movie, we become reacquainted with our partner's mind and body on an ongoing basis. We recover curiosity for the unseen ways our partner is changing in front of our eyes.

Like Carla and Miguel, Gina and Elizabeth had spent nearly two decades in the familiarity trance. They were so busy with their business and taking care of their eleven-year-old daughter that they rarely had time for sex. They laughed at my suggestion to "see fresh," but this simple exercise turned out to be a game changer for the couple and renewed their sexual spark. I also encouraged them to go outside the well-etched tracks of their familiar routines and take new paths during sex. At home, I suggested they nurture each other more because they had become used to interacting like business partners rather than lovers.

When we met six weeks later, Gina and Elizabeth were a different couple. I wondered what accounted for the lighthearted flirting that I was witnessing between them. Both women began speaking, then paused, and graciously offered the other the lead. Gina accepted: "We were skeptical when we left your office that things could be as good or better than they were in the early days, but that evening Elizabeth offered to brush my hair before bed rather than falling asleep on the sofa. She used to brush my hair when we first got together, but I thought those days were over."

"I felt so much tenderness from Elizabeth that I started moving toward sex. Elizabeth stopped me, which was surprising and intriguing at the same time. I felt like she was playing hard to get when she is the one who usually presses *me* for sex. Elizabeth asked me to remove my robe, and I obliged, though I felt oddly shy. She looked at me for a long time and put her head on my belly like she used to do before our daughter was born. It was so tender that I began to weep. That night we snuggled all night long."

Gina continues with the story: "The next morning, we kissed for a while and then I pushed Elizabeth's head to my crotch, but she didn't taste me. Instead, she began describing my genitals like they were a work of art. I could feel currents of energy going down to my toes when her hand grazed my vulva. I had never felt anything like it. It was like having sex without being sexual, but it was very intense. That experience opened something in me. I felt a renewed sense of trust and appreciation for Elizabeth; like after all these years, we could find each other again."

If you think these stories are too good to be true, I have news for you: you already have a wonderful partner too—you just forgot to notice. "Wonder" and curiosity are both inextricably linked. As we become curious about who is here now, beneath the petrified roles of day-to-day living, we can experience the wonder of novelty with our long-term partner regularly.

Elizabeth now takes a turn at reporting: "Last week, Gina rubbed my feet as she often does while we watch television. This time, she put on some music and blindfolded me. I had no idea what was happening, but I completely surrendered." Gina jumps in again, "I made rubbing Elizabeth's feet a mindful touch exercise where I let myself stay curious and exploratory. I became intensely engaged with merely feeling the texture of her skin, including the crevices between her toes." "Afterward, we had some of the hottest sex we ever had," says Elizabeth, "even though we were both exhausted. I have to say that I never thought I would feel this way again. It's like I'm with Gina and with someone new."

When we are enchanted in stage 1, we don't have to work to be present because novelty draws us to each other like iron to a magnet. Because of novelty and our heightened arousal, we are naturally more present. We notice intimate details about the shape of our beloved's fingers and wrists. We record facial expressions that convey disappointment or delight. These details are mesmerizing because they are new. Eventually, we lose sight of the details, relying instead on impressions we formed at an earlier time. Wayne Dyer reminds us, "If you change the way you look at things, the things you look at change."[37] Instead of seeing the "same old thing," we can see fresh.

Try this now: Shift your attention from what I am saying to how the words appear on the page. Give yourself a good couple of minutes to pay close attention to the shape and size of the letters and the thickness of the paper. Imagine you are from another planet that doesn't have books.

You don't know what this object is for, only that it has unidentifiable symbols. Smell and touch the paper, the spine, front, back, and sides of this book. What are you noticing about the book now that you didn't see before?

We can do this "seeing fresh" practice with our partner, who unlike a book, is changing every day. Greg Johanson, a founding trainer of the Hakomi Institute, writes that "humility" rather than "certainty" helps us find each other again.[38] With mindfulness, we delete the cache and listen, look, and touch freshly. We can train our eyes to look for novelty in familiar places and, in so doing, recover our curiosity again and again.

Through erotic presence, the ordinary becomes extraordinary because we are *here* to enjoy it. If the inner observer's eyes are open, we can also see our habits in real time, particularly those that diminish our PEP. Befriending our natural eroticism through mindfulness and mindful touch makes the cultivation of novelty an "inside job," and helps us access our PEP more regularly.

## MINDFUL ACTIVITIES AND NAKED REFLECTIONS

. . . . . . . . . . . . . . . . . . . . . . . . . . . . . . . . . . . . . . . . . . . . . . . . . . . . . . . . . . . . . . .

## Seeing Fresh

. . . . . . . . . . . . . . . . . . . . . . . . . . . . . . . . . . . . . . . . . . . . . . . . . . . . . . . . . . . . . . .

Seeing fresh is an exercise to train attention and cultivate a state of novelty. It is a lifelong practice to overcome the familiarity trance by meeting for the first time, again and again. To do this, we must delete our preconceptions, expectations, and internal models about our partner and take them in as if we were meeting a stranger. Eventually, we can bring the same practice into the bedroom. We can meet freshly, letting wonder and curiosity guide our actions.

### Part 1 (2 minutes)

1. Begin by sitting across from your partner.
2. Close your eyes and create a mental image of your partner.
3. Then, think about the ways this person is predictable, all the

features you know so well, including their expressions, habits, and preferences, even the things that annoy you.

4. Notice the state this mental activity creates in you.

## Part 2 (2 minutes)

1. Open your eyes and notice how your partner looks to you from this "familiarity state."
2. Only see what you expect to see, with little to no curiosity about this person. Just be aware of all of the details that you already know.
3. Notice your level of engagement. What happens inside of you as you do this? How attractive is this person to you right now?

## Part 3 (2 minutes)

1. Close your eyes and empty again. Let go of all of your associations, preconceptions, and judgments about this person. Imagine you have a way of deleting everything you "know" about this person.
2. Find the part of you that can be open and curious. Sense how you do that. If being curious was a state of mind, how can you create a "curiosity state" instead of a "familiarity state"? One way is to have humility rather than certainty. Imagine that every day the world is born anew, and your partner is different every time you meet.
3. Pretend you are about to meet the person in front of you for the very first time.

## Part 4 (5 minutes)

1. Open your eyes and see fresh. Look for newness.
2. First focus on what you see rather than what you imagine to be there. Be curious and look for details, such as colors, wrinkles, shapes, and so on. What do you notice when you see fresh?
3. Go a bit deeper now, taking in not just this person's physical features, but something about what you see behind their face: their energy, spirit, and heart. What kind of a being is this? What do you sense in this "one and only" meeting about this person's hopes and fears?

*Part 5 (2 minutes)*

1. If it feels safe for you to do so, imagine this is not only the first but also the last time you will see this person (one day, this will be true).
2. What opens up in you? What is your impulse toward this person?
3. Either follow this impulse or notice anything that stops you from expressing this impulse.

## Naked Reflections

After the exercise is over, take some time to talk to each other about the activity. Here are some conversation starters:

Were you able to see fresh?
What shift did you make to do that?
What did you notice that you hadn't seen before?
What were you curious about?
What was your impulse?
Did anything stop you from following your impulse?
What would it be like to bring this same "curious humility" to the bedroom? To see, meet, and touch fresh?

## Mindful Touch

This exercise helps to develop curiosity and erotic presence. One person touches, and one person receives, with both focused on exploration and pleasure. The person who is touching practices bringing interest and presence to the connection without trying to arouse their partner or prepare for sexual activity. For the receiver, the focus is on practicing nonjudging awareness of sensation (i.e., avoiding labeling sensations as pleasant and unpleasant). Notice the different qualities of sensation at the point of contact and in other parts of your body.

Decide ahead of time:

1. Who will be partner A, the toucher, and who will be partner B, the receiver.
2. How long you will do this activity. You can start with 5 minutes each way, building up to 20 minutes, or more if you enjoy it.
3. What part of the body you will each explore.

## Step 1

Both partners spend 5 minutes in mindfulness, sitting across from one another. This activity might involve turning awareness inside to feel your body or studying the rhythm and accompanying sensations of the breath. Bring your attention back to your breath every time your mind wanders. You can also try doing these things while softly gazing at your partner.

## Step 2 (5 minutes or longer)

Partner A, the toucher: Explore a part of your partner's body physically as if you haven't seen it before (cheek, leg, thigh, stomach, arms, or back—not genitals). Make sure you have permission before getting started. Begin by gently resting your hand on the area to allow your partner to get used to the contact. Don't try to second-guess what your partner might like. Go with how you feel and follow your impulses.

Stay curious: Explore the landscape (texture, ridges, temperature) of your partner's body. Be aware of the sensations in your fingers and palm. Also, notice the rest of your body as you make contact with your partner. Let this activity be about your pleasure and exploration rather than performance. Meet this body for the first time.

Bring presence: Instead of trying to arouse your partner, you want to communicate your presence through touch. Direct your attention to the point of contact between your fingertip and your partner's skin. Observe your partner's responses, such as changes in skin tone, breath, sound, and so on.

Pause, and bring your attention back to the moment whenever you get swept up into thinking, any discomfort arises, or you are disengaging or becoming automatic. Either stop the activity or wait for a fresh impulse to appear before resuming.

Partner B, the person being touched: Tune into the experience and focus on receiving rather than becoming aroused. Bring your awareness to the point of contact between your skin and your partner's fingertip. Notice sensations in the area of the contact. Notice sensations in other parts of your body. If you feel aroused, telescope in on the feelings that accompany arousal; find words to describe the sensation. Pause, or discontinue the exercise if the sensation becomes unpleasant or you find yourself dissociating.

After you have completed the agreed time each way, share your observations.

. . . . . . . . . . . . . . . . . . . . . . . . . . . . . . . . . . . . . . . . . . . . . . . . . . . . . . . . . .

## Naked Reflections
. . . . . . . . . . . . . . . . . . . . . . . . . . . . . . . . . . . . . . . . . . . . . . . . . . . . . . . . . .

Were you able to bring erotic presence to the touch activity? If so, how did you do that? If not, what got in the way?

What sensations did you notice as both giver and receiver?

As the giver, what did you notice in your partner as you were touching? What did you observe in yourself?

Which is more comfortable—giving or receiving?

As the receiver, how do you react when the touch isn't quite right? How do you manage activation if you have some?

What habits, patterns, or emotional reactions did you notice in either role?

# 3.

## EROTIC COOPERATION

### Holding Hands through the Hard Stuff

Many of us believe that great sex is the result of good chemistry. Still, no amount of chemistry will prepare you for differences that will likely arise in your erotic preferences and levels of desire over time. Neither chemistry—nor love, for that matter—will spare you from illness, disability, aging, and general life stress, all of which affect partner sex. Life only becomes more complex and, consequently, more stressful as we journey together.

Despite these certainties, working with couples has shown me how much effort it takes for partners to hold erotic struggles with their hands clasped together. Harder still, for each to expose the very things they want to hide or deny. However, if we're going to take the naked path together, we must travel as cooperative allies. Otherwise, we will bicker all along the way. Teamwork is the heart of awakened intimacy and the fruit of erotic cooperation.

While we may worry that running into difficulties is a sign that something is wrong with us or that our relationship is doomed, it could very well mean that love is working its magic. At stage 1, love and desire flow between you because there is an opening for them. This very openness also exposes each person's "deepest, darkest wounds, their desperation and mistrust, and their rawest emotional trigger points," claims John Welwood.[1]

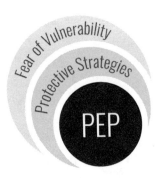

FIGURE 3.1 CHAPTER 3 PEP BARRIERS

When unhealed wounds or new fears surface, many people engage in protective patterns that snuff out their loving feelings and inhibit growth. They close the door to their hearts and bar the sexual gates. Although this course is typical, Welwood offers an alternative: "When two partners with a deep bond choose to work with the obstacles arising between them, this deepens their connection with themselves and each other, and can provide a mutual sense of path and direction."[2]

We step onto the naked path when we realize as individuals that we can't escape our past hurts and agree to use our relationship for healing and growth. Awakened intimacy involves meeting yourself and your partner beneath layers of defensiveness to find the tender, compassionate, and resilient ground of your being. When we connect to that potential in ourselves, it becomes possible to stop blaming each other for our struggles and to face our problems with hands clasped.

## OUR MOSAIC SELVES

> A person is a fluid process, not a fixed and static entity; a flowing river of change, not a block of solid material.
> —Carl Rogers[3]

As we move through life together, we go in and out of a variety of states. We fluctuate between being open and contracted, loving and fearful. In extreme situations, we can go into warlike states.[4] Each state has a neural profile established over time through repetition.[5] When these different profiles switch on, we may seem like different people, which is why we can think of our states as "parts" of ourselves that emerge in different contexts.

It is easy to see that you are more a mosaic of parts than a unified self by remembering the times you have said, "One part of me wants X, and another part of me wants Y." Moreover, each state/part "contains within it an emerging story, often with rules and more readily accessible memory (explicit and implicit)."[6] For example, we may feel dejected if our partner is late from work and doesn't call home. In our "dejected state," we remember other times when the people in our life "forgot about us," gathering evidence that supports the felt sense that we are unimportant.

In response, our body slumps, and we start to feel worthless. To protect ourselves from such feelings, we may become aggrieved and go on the offensive. When our partner explains that they witnessed a fatal accident and stopped to give a police report, our dejection quickly shifts to concern. Now, in our "concerned state," we think of those less fortunate than ourselves, who have lost someone they love. No longer in our orginal dejected state, we are merely happy that our partner is home safe, no matter the hour.

While love can pull forward our best self (remember the line from *Jerry McGuire*: "You make me want to be a better man"?),[7] it can also unleash a surprising beast. When triggered, we may yell, threaten to leave, become cold, critical, or demeaning. In all likelihood, the way you act in your war state is not how you act with friends or in the workplace.

To see what I mean, recall a recent conflict with your partner. How did you behave? Think back to how you looked, including your body posture and facial expressions. What about your tone of voice? Would your work colleagues, who know you to be reasonable and even-tempered, be surprised to see this other part of you?

This changeability from one state to another can lead us to wonder, am I Jekyll or Hyde? Is my "true" self when I feel strong and self-confident, or is it the sad, abandoned me who feels rejected and unwanted? Am I forgiving or full of complaints? Although we may prefer some states over others, the naked path is all-partisan. "The dark thought, the shame, the malice, meet them at the door laughing and invite them in," wrote the thirteenth-century Persian poet Rumi.[8] For we can only be intimate with ourselves when we welcome all of our states/parts, especially the ones we'd rather not see.

By now, your partner knows all of your states, which is another way that intimate relationships are naked. Consequently, the enchantment we feel at stage 3 is qualitatively different from the charm that befalls us at stage 1. We are not swept away or blinded by desire. We see our partner's humanness, including the flaws. Nor are we trying to establish a pain-free relationship. Our enchantment at stage 3 is with the *process* of conscious relating. We are on a course to become more wakeful and whole by transforming the barriers to our pure erotic potential. Chief among them is the fear of vulnerability.

Not only does your partner know your states, but your partner affects your states as well. You might notice how you react when your partner comes home in a foul mood. Do the good feelings you had until that moment dissolve at once? What about when your partner is thrilled to see you? As mammals, our capacity to "feel with" each other can be regulating or dysregulating. If we are particularly sensitive to "emotion contagion," we will catch every bad mood around us.[9] We will get angry in response to our partner's anger or tense when our partner gets tense.

Some of the states we go into during conflicts are "legacy states" that hearken back to childhood. They involve feeling helpless, unloved, terrified, overwhelmed, powerless, or worthless and are associated with our early wounding. Such states are hard to bear because they are so dysregulating and painful. Thus, we employ defensive maneuvers to avoid them. We may get loud or sarcastic to get our partner to back off, or we may shut down or withdraw. These protective strategies, in turn, prevent you from being in a naked exchange with eros and with your partner. Consequently, they, too, become a barrier to your PEP.

We don't make up our protective strategies on the spot. We learn these behaviors out of necessity when we're young and particularly vulnerable. Unfortunately, the ways we now protect against vulnerability can also prevent us from having what we want. For instance, blaming our partners may cause them to retreat when we most want their care. Moreover, our strategies may keep us from falling into legacy states at the moment, but they don't resolve the underlying issue. We are no less reactive the next time our partner does something that triggers us. Thus, when we defend against vulnerability, we can't heal or grow.

We can start on the path toward becoming more wakeful and loving by engaging with these questions as a daily practice:

How do we love our partners as they are, even when they go into protective states?

How do we work with *ourselves* when we feel hurt, shocked, confused or angry, instead of blaming our partner?

How can we shift from defense to compassion for ourselves and our partners?

We may choose to "live the questions now" as Rilke put it,[10] as opposed to seeing our difficulties as wrong and trying to "fix" them. By developing awareness and compassion, the heart can grow wings, which is how you can use the issues that are dividing you to become deeply connected.

## THE IMPASSE

Have you ever gotten into an argument that didn't resolve? Did the problem become only more entrenched as you tried to address it? This experience is so universal that many couples decide to "agree to disagree." Others get stuck in never-ending loops that suck the life out of their relationship erotically and emotionally.

What contributes to this kind of standoff? In intimate relationships, we are usually reacting to our partners' protective states or parts more than their position. The mannerisms, words, and facial expressions that our partners use to avoid experiencing their legacy states triggers *our* legacy states. Our legacy states trigger our protective patterns, which in turn, triggers theirs, ad infinitum.

In the second segment of our Passion and Presence retreats, we dive into each couple's most stubborn interaction patterns, commonly referred to as the "impasse." No one looks forward to this. They arrive as if attending their funeral. Remarkably, over the weekend, the same couples who came gripped with anxiety, leave with soft open faces and hearts brimming with compassion. How? By engaging in experiences that reveal the deep-seated vulnerabilities at the core of their conflicts, they recover a renewed sense of hope for their relationship.

Eric and Max came to one of my retreats as a last-ditch effort to turn their sexless marriage around. Both were ready to end their relationship unless something shifted dramatically. Max, a safety engineer from Encinitas, California, plants himself in the chair in the session room as if he has no intention of ever leaving. By contrast, Eric, a general partner of a venture capital firm, is leaning forward, jiggling spare change in his pocket. He appears to be ready for takeoff.

When I ask how I can support their erotic life Max doesn't hesitate. He tells me he feels pressured by Eric's constant appeals for sex. Eric responds defensively and charges Max with abusing his veto power. He asks me if it is fair to withhold sex from your partner indefinitely. I refrain from answering the question and instead contact Eric's feelings of powerlessness and frustration.

While all couples have some version of the impasse, or "stuck place," a conflict around the frequency of sex is perhaps the most common one. In this impasse, the so-called high desire partner makes bids for sex that are refused by the so-called low desire partner.[11] The increasingly "sex-starved" partner feels deprived and rejected and becomes ever more insistent on having sex. The low desire partner feels pressured and in turn, rigidly refuses. The push-pull of their approach-withdrawal dynamic polarizes their positions, even though they may not be as far apart as it seems.

My first step is to help this couple feel safe with me. I validate Max's need to be in a place of choice and Eric's experience of abandonment when Max pushes him away. I add that there are likely good reasons for the positions they are holding and that we can use our time together to discover something new about this painful standoff. I also reassure them that no one has to change because acceptance is a core feature of a mindful approach.

I then ask Max to tell me what Eric does to express his interest in having sex. "He grabs my cock," Max says hotly. Eric says, "You used to like it when I did that," practically rising from his seat. Max rolls his eyes and sighs with exasperation. "Well, newsflash, I don't anymore." He flicks his hand and turns away.

"Try being a bit smugger," Eric suggests sarcastically, then shifts tactics. "Oh, what's the point of arguing, I don't have time for this." His legs are shaking restlessly. "That's right, your time is so 'precious,'" Max says, making finger quotes when he says "precious." "See," Max says, turning to me, "all Eric wants is to 'screw and run.'" "See," Eric counters, shaking his head. "Max is impossible to talk to." Eric gestures, "What's the use?" and falls back against his chair.

Scientists and communication theorists have been studying these self-reinforcing loops since the 1940s.[12] Variously called "demon dialogues,"[13] "the more, the more,"[14] the "negativity cycle,"[15] "vulnerability cycle,"[16] or the "reciprocal interaction loop" (RIL),[17] these vicious cycles only leave couples on opposing teams, caught in deadlocks.

Michele Sheinkman and Mona Fishbane, who call these loops the "vulnerability cycle," write, "While caught up in one of these impasses, the partners are unable to empathize and see the other's perspective. They feel offended and violated by the other's behavior, and become increasingly defensive, disconnected, and entangled in power struggles and misunderstandings."[18]

Sadly, by the time many couples enter therapy, it is often too late. Couples' therapists try, often in vain, to stop the hemorrhaging out of goodwill, hope, and compassion between partners that started months or perhaps years earlier. Many interventions only ensure that verbal jabs do not puncture vital organs. Trying to solve the problem by looking at who "started" it only makes things worse. The communication is circular. It could theoretically go on till eternity. Instead, we must "jump out of the system" and look at the pattern itself.[19]

## PROTECTORS IGNITE PROTECTORS

Does your jaw tighten when you are kept waiting, or your partner leaves dishes in the sink—again! Many of us can go from zero to one hundred very quickly, reacting with an intensity that is disproportionate to the crime.[20] Our blood pressure rises, our chest tightens, and our stomach churns when our partner enters the room. In turn, our partner reacts to our micro-expressions, voice tone, and overt displays of aggression or disappointment. Such behaviors can trigger a cascade of stress hormones that ready us for quick action.[21]

While we like to think we have free will, much of our behavior is programmed and predictable. For instance, your partner knows how you will shrug your shoulder and sigh when you are frustrated, and you know how they will glaze over when you say you want to talk. Such response patterns become interlocking and eventually, hyper-stable. We sometimes experience this stability as "being stuck."

When we are in our vicious cycle, we are reacting from our emotional brain. A perceived danger trips the threat response, and we attack or retreat through stonewalling, shutting down, or leaving. Even if we are not loud and aggressive, the pattern of perceived danger and defense keeps repeating because of tracks laid down in the brain, explains Mona Fishbane, the author of *Loving with the Brain in Mind*.[22] Over time, the sense of inevitability—of being unable to stop the escalation—can set in. We feel stuck and helpless to break the loop despite our feelings of shame and regret afterward.[23]

This inability to stop the cycle is not only demoralizing; it is also hazardous to our health.[24] Our nervous system stays on high alert, and our body responds as if we are living in a war zone—and the experience that we are living in one is "real" to us. Automatic reactivity is also hazardous to your relationship. Marion Solomon and Stan Tatkin, the authors of *Love and War in Intimate Relationships*, caution that when couples develop a fast-reacting interaction style without repair, goodwill erodes very quickly.[25]

## Why Do We React So Fast?

While we may chalk up our impasse to a case of irreconcilable differences, what drives the negativity loop is commonly fear. Humans have endured as a species by honing their survival instincts. We scan for safety and danger regularly using a neurobiological mechanism called "neuroception."[26] Just as dogs go on high alert when other dogs walk by, humans can go from loving to teeth baring in a flash.

This threat response explains why we can so quickly go from loving to hating.

Under threat, the higher brain centers shut down our reasoning abilities, and we are unable to inhibit the amygdala and the hypothalamic-pituitary-adrenal (HPA) axis, our stress-response system. Without input from the prefrontal cortex, we act without thinking. We jump from a snake that is only a rope, for example, because our emotional memory contains the knowledge that low moving, wiggling objects can be deadly.[27]

Likewise, the gestures our partner makes when we're in our negative loop can resemble danger signs from our past. For instance, the look our father made before he became violent, or the cold shoulder we got when we disappointed our mother. When we see something that is "similar enough," we automatically protect ourselves from this dangerous threat.[28]

Over the years, I've seen many behaviors that trigger protective states. If we had a video recording of these actions, we might see these kinds of things in one or both partners: body turned away, clipped voice, yelling, eyebrows raised, throwing up hands, exasperated sighs, bodily collapse, reddened face, silence, pouting, pinched expression, set jaw, expansive chest, hard eyes, fake smile, lack of eye contact, arms folded, hands in fists, rigid spine, glazed eyes, stony silence, and statements that begin with, "you always," or "you never."

We can classify these behaviors as evidence of fight-flight-freeze mechanisms. Deb Dana, a clinician and consultant specializing in working with complex trauma, uses the image of a ladder to explain the neurophysiological states that are part of our regulatory system.[29] At the top of the ladder, we are in what neuroscientist Stephan Porges calls our "social engagement system."[30] Here, we feel relaxed, safe, and optimistic, because our ventral vagal nerve communes with our parasympathetic nervous system to calm us down. When we go into fight-or-flight mode, we move down a rung on the ladder. The sympathetic nervous system switches on, and we become action oriented and combative.

We also have a shutdown system, orchestrated by the dorsal vagal nerve. When Eric collapses into the chair and says, "What's the use," he loses all sense of fight and becomes withdrawn and nonverbal. When we shut down—rather than calm down—we go two rungs below social engagement. In this state, the world looks dark and desolate; we feel hopeless and alone.

We can learn to use the inner observer to disidentify from extreme states so that we can regulate ourselves more quickly. Then, instead of guarding our vulnerability, we can move out of our survival positions and into a connected state by revealing the feelings we are safeguarding so fiercely.

## THE RECIPROCAL INTERACTION LOOP (RIL)

Albert Einstein famously said, "We cannot solve our problems with the same level of thinking that created them."[31] It is for this reason that we must rise above our programming when we are in the low of a deadlock. We need self-regulation tools to climb up the ladder and a meta-perspective to disidentify from our protective states (refer to figure 2.2, "Disidentification"). Of all the models I have looked at to help couples do this, I have found the reciprocal interaction loop (RIL) diagramming process to be the most effective. The tool was developed by Halko Weiss to help two people get to the core of their conflicts very quickly and also to shift states.[32]

The activity begins by working with a specific conflict and then listing the overt behaviors of each partner's "protector" part or state. In other words, how do partners come across to each other during the argument? The next step is to mindfully study the hidden legacy state these protectors are protecting, along with the legacy states and protective behaviors they evoke in the other.

Let's return to Max and Eric:

When Max flicks his hand and turns away, it triggers a legacy state in Eric. Eric sounds superior when he says: "I don't have time for this," but underneath he is starting to feel powerless and tossed away (one of his legacy states). Eric's protective behaviors, in turn, trigger a legacy state in Max. Max feels unimportant and stupid, which he defends against by

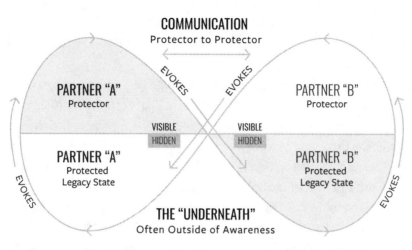

**FIGURE 3.2 RECIPROCAL INTERACTION LOOP**

When partner A's protector triggers partner B's legacy state, partner B's protector comes to the rescue. In turn, partner B's protector triggers partner A's legacy state, and partner A's protector comes to the rescue. In the loop, communication is between protectors. Both partners are unaware of the hidden legacy state they are protecting, and they do not see their partner's vulnerability.

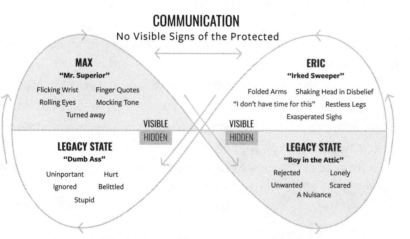

**FIGURE 3.3 THE RIL DIAGRAMMING PROCESS**

This process involves listing the qualities of each partner's protector state and giving it a name. Then, each partner explores the hidden feelings their partner's protector triggers in them. The final step is to name these legacy states and explore how our protector and protected parts interact and reinforce each other when we're at an impasse.

rolling his eyes and saying, "See, all Eric wants to do is 'screw and run.'" Unless one of them calls a truce, the loop of vulnerability, threat, and defense will go on forever.

Weiss uses the symbol of the infinity sign (∞) with arrows to illustrate the way Max's protector evokes Eric's legacy state (the protected), which in turn evokes Eric's protector, which in turn evokes Max's legacy state (the protected), which in turn evokes Max's protector (see figure 3.2, "Reciprocal Interaction Loop"). By diagramming the RIL together, Max and Eric recognize how their attempts to resolve their struggles only perpetuate the loop. They generate names for their protector and protected states as they gain an understanding of the underlying legacy states hidden behind their "protectors" (see figure 3.3, "The RIL Diagramming Process").

Each state or part comes with a distinct set of emotions, sensations, and view of life.[33] When caught in their RIL, Max and Eric selectively remember other times they felt "stupid" or "rejected." The feelings and body sensations that accompany such moments seem like an unbroken stream, a continuous "reality" rather than a transient state. On the ground level, we take our state-bound feelings and perceptions as the truth. The sky view allows us to "rise" above our programming and shift from adversaries to allies.

Eric and Max now see this moment for what it is for each of them—a state-induced dynamic, accompanied by an old, automatic response. Max concedes that when he is in his protector state he forgets how loving and supportive Eric can be. When we disidentify from protective states, we transform the feelings of hurt, fear, and blame that block us from intimate contact into appreciation and care.

## FROM STALEMATE TO "SOUL MATE"

A true soul mate is probably the most important person you'll ever meet, because they tear down your walls and smack you awake.
—Elizabeth Gilbert[34]

If we are honest with ourselves, we fancy a partner who is always kind, interested, and encouraging, a partner who can attune to our need for closeness or space, and recognize when we want practical guidance or physical holding, a partner who is ready for sex when we are, and who also wants to do it "our" way—in other words, except for the sex part, the parent we never had. The popular image of the soul mate captures this: our "perfect partner" is what we all want.

It is because love relationships recreate so many of the conditions of early childhood that we enter into them with hopes of receiving the care and protection we needed as children. Some therapists assert that intimate partners can and should provide one another with the safety, attunement, and support that grow children into secure adults.[35] Indeed, a warm, nurturing connection can anchor us at any stage of life, not just when we take our first wobbly steps upright. For example, studies show that the healing effect of psychotherapy is mostly due to the relationship between client and therapist and not to a particular method or technique.[36]

While human beings help each other grow, they also hurt each other. In intimate relationships, in particular, these two forces go tête-à-tête. Thus, there will no doubt be times when your partner is unwilling or unable to meet your needs. Sometimes the pain we feel when this happens links to our childhood wounds.

As children, we may have received something unwanted, even toxic—like abuse, criticism, or overcontrol. Or we may not have gotten the care and understanding we dearly needed. As a result, we may have sensitivities with regard to feeling seen, heard, attended to, or respected. "When two people fall in love, the seeds of later conflicts are already present," claim Solomon and Tatkin. "Both carry their personal history wired into their brains, and these neural networks are waiting to be activated by reminders of early attachment failures."[37]

In our relationship, the pain we experience when our partner is distracted or impatient may remind us of the many times we were disregarded or treated brusquely as children. We may, in turn, experience intense feelings of hurt and despair, even rage. In response, our first instinct is to try to change our partner so we can stop hurting. Unfortunately, this usually only leads to more hurt and despair, which was evident between Eric and Max.

As adults, growth sometimes happens best when we are left frustrated and dissatisfied in some way. For it is at this point of deep disappointment that we can see more clearly and compassionately our needy and hurt inner child. It is also when we can help that part of us grow up. When we encounter the familiar feeling of emptiness that Welwood claims "we have been trying to fill with relationships all of our life,"[38] our disappointment becomes an ally. However, for this to be possible, we must bring the warmth and acceptance we want from our partner to ourselves. It is as simple and, yes, as hard, as that.

Many of us have walled our hearts off because the pain we experienced in our youth was too big to bear. We may not know that we now have adult capacities to feel and heal our hurt parts. The naked path shows us that we do. Romantic yearnings notwithstanding, a soul mate is not your twin or better half. A soul mate helps you evolve your potential by challenging you to cultivate capacities that may not have taken root in childhood. However, this ripening doesn't occur by being in synch with your every wish or protecting you from pain.

Does this mean we should give up on wanting love and kindness from our partner? The answer is no. Stage 3 couples typically experience an abundance of love because they impose fewer conditions on the amount and kind of love they receive. On the naked path, it is, in fact, for the sake of love that we give up wanting love to fulfill our unfillable needs and desires. We stop blaming each other and look *inside* for the source of our pain. When we view our reactivity as an opportunity to heal and grow we are finally able to hold hands through the hard stuff.

## FINDING OUR WINGS OF AWARENESS AND COMPASSION

It may surprise you to learn that we need to tolerate peace to develop a cooperative relationship. Peace doesn't mean we never fight. It means we come back into loving connection after we do. For this to happen, we must work with our fears of being intimate and vulnerable, instead of using our protector parts to distance ourselves from our partner.

The felt sense of being "in this together" as undefended allies may be strange to you. If the home environment you grew up in was full of strife, a relationship that features yelling, or cold silences might seem more natural than supporting each other under stress. You may even have the habit of generating conflict to get it over with, feeling anxious about the "calm before the storm."

To sustain a loving relationship, we must increase our capacity to bear the discomfort of unfamiliar ways of experiencing relationships. And over time, increase our ability to move toward those "new" states. At stage 3, we train ourselves to take the neurological "high road," of being reflective and aware, rather than reactive under stress.[39] However, despite our best intentions, the high road will sometimes be blocked to us, and we will find ourselves triggered automatically.

It is for this very reason that stage 3 couples bring a mindful tool kit on the journey to their PEP. They take measures to maintain their (internal) shock absorbers, headlights, and brake pads because the terrain is bumpy for stretches and the weather uncertain. In cases of flooding, or when the engine blows a gasket, we can use a four-step process I created called PREP as emergency roadside assistance (see figure 3.4, "PREP Process").

## THE PREP PROCESS

Step 1, **pause**, is turning off the ignition. The engine has to cool down before we can open the hood.

Step 2, **regulate**, is how we let the hot air evaporate before charging at the engine to see what is wrong. Until we are in ventral vagal, and our prefrontal cortex is back online, we cannot bring goodwill to the situation.

Step 3, **explore**, involves opening the hood and inspecting the engine to see what our protector is protecting.

Step 4, **peaceful presence**, is how we care for each part of the engine; we don't yank out parts or kick the engine for having trouble.

Let's look in more detail at each step.

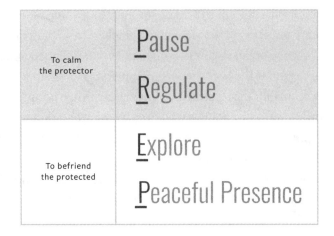

| | |
|---|---|
| To calm the protector | P̲ause<br><br>R̲egulate |
| To befriend the protected | E̲xplore<br><br>P̲eaceful Presence |

**FIGURE 3.4 PREP PROCESS**

The PREP process serves as emergency roadside assistance when we are unable to take the "high road" of awareness and reflection. The four steps show us how to interrupt our reactivity and explore whatever is driving our protective behaviors.

## Step 1: Pause

The way we react to stress goes back to our early life and relationships with primary caretakers.[40] Depending on which genes switched on, we may have a quiet nervous system, or we may be a "hot reactor."[41] Robert Sapolsky tells us that in any given species, at least 20 percent of its members see threat even when there isn't any. Likewise, those with trauma histories, or high resting baseline levels of sympathetic nervous system (SNS) activity, may naturally be more reactive.

Arousal is a good thing when it supports vitality and engagement, as well as sexual response, but too much activation can be dysregulating. As we increase our sense of resilience, we can recover from fear-induced arousal spikes quickly, helping us regain a calmer and emotionally regulated state.[42] Unfortunately, when our "primitives" hijack us, as Stan Tatkin calls the warmongering reactive parts of the brain, we lose these capacities.[43] At such times, a mindful pause can function as a circuit breaker. It interrupts the outpouring of stress hormones that readies us for quick action.

One of the purported benefits of regular mindfulness practice is that it increases response flexibility, which helps us consider our choices rather than act out automatically.[44] When we have space between our feelings and actions, we see options that can help us be more loving, creative, and responsive. In other words, a resilient nervous system enables us to be emotionally intelligent.

## Step 2: Regulate

While we may want our partners to take back their unkind words and soothe us, it is essential to realize that they, no doubt, are struggling too. In such instances, we have to put on our oxygen mask first. As we all know by now, we can't negotiate with a fire-breathing dragon or domineering dictator. These internal protector parts are warriors; they care only about self-preservation. To recover a spirit of goodwill, we must wait for the arrival of our "ambassadors," to borrow another term from Tatkin.[45] These are the rational parts of ourselves that prefer to make love rather than war.

So how can we get into our resilience zone as we PREP? We can build a collection of practices to help us regulate, regain calmness, and bounce back so that we have them at hand when we need them.[46] Deb Dana calls resilience practices ventral vagal anchors.[47] We can anchor by creating "reset moments" through practices that have a scientific basis in how our bodies—our physiologies—work. The easiest solo practice is the deep exhale, where we sigh deeply. Another is to evoke a memory in which we felt safe and at ease, and to breathe this in. We can also walk in nature, exercise, or listen to music that we love.

Daniel Goleman and Richard Davidson claim that meditation can be extremely regulating even if we've struggled for years to feel safe and calm.[48] Moreover, studies show that mindfulness slows the release of the stress hormone cortisol during a conflict.[49] However, if we use the time we are "mindful" to justify our actions, we are ramping up the defense system. To calm the turbulence in our nervous system, we must stay with our felt experience and avoid creating a story to justify our position.

## Step 3: Explore

> There is one non-negotiable ticket for admission to creating and sustaining intimate partnerships: the understanding that what we are experiencing in a relationship is a reflection of our own internal state of being. This means inquiring into each thought, feeling, and behavior with the recognition that our emotional reactions can best tell us something about ourselves, rather than about our partners.
> —Jett Psaris and Marlena S. Lyons[50]

It can be especially difficult to apply mindfulness to our relationships, but our person-to-person interactions are often what benefit from mindful practice the most. There are numerous stories of cave-dwelling yogis who lose their peaceful state the moment they interact with human beings. Inevitably, we will experience similar agitation through daily contact with those closest to us if we have buttons to push—which we all do. While that sounds like terrible news, the truth is that we can only heal wounds that are visible in this way, and we may do so through mindfully turning our attention to them when they arise.

As we saw, we all have a particular sensitivity. Perhaps yours is centered around feeling controlled. Alternatively, maybe you are sensitive to feeling belittled, criticized, abandoned, or manipulated. Although these "vulnerabilities" often grow out of our family of origin, they may also derive from power inequities or sociocultural traumas such as discrimination, poverty, marginalization, violence, social dislocation, or war-related experiences.[51] When our sensitivity is triggered and we feel like a traumatic experience is happening to us—again—our reactions can be extreme.

Weiss likes to say that when our protector shows up, something needs our protection.[52] To locate the protected, we have to slow down to feel what is happening underneath our protector. Then, we can mine for the deeper and more vulnerable parts of our experience. These parts are usually invisible even to *us*.

To explore, we use the skill of mindful self-study, which involves directing attention toward the unpleasant emotion or sensation that accompanies the activation.[53] To see what is driving our protective behaviors, we must also be willing to touch into the helplessness, grief, confusion, or fear—whatever pain our protector is trying to prevent us from feeling—in an open, curious way. This open stance allows new information to emerge from the depths of our being. The longer we linger, the more information emerges. Sometimes memories surface, sometimes we get only a general understanding of our wounded part.

Here are some things we might investigate in mindfulness:

What kind of state is this?
What emotions come along with this?
What is my body expressing in this state?
How old do I feel right now?
What earlier situation seems connected to this state?
What am I expecting as I protect myself like this?

When Eric engaged in mindful self-study after a flare-up with Max, he noticed that his muscles were very tight and that he felt a sense of pressure behind his skull. Eventually, the pressure seemed to connect to a sense of urgency, a feeling like he would have to move fast or lose out on something. This sense of "losing out" led to an underlying feeling of being rejected and alone. He saw an image of his protected part, which he called "The boy in the attic," and his heart softened when he felt the boy's pain.

At stage 3, we dive deeply, continuously, whether our partner does so or not. Yes, our partner was undoubtedly reactive, too, but a mindful approach involves investigating the feelings inside of *you*. There's always another level underneath, something we haven't discovered yet. When Eric realized that he was feeling rejected and alone, he understood why his protector was working so hard for him. Typically, when we get some understanding of the protected, we experience a surge of sadness or grief, and a simultaneous letting go. A knot unfurls, and our heart opens again.

## Step 4: Peaceful Presence to Ourselves

Cupid is a champion for love—both for us and for others. When we have a good relationship with all of our parts—protected and protector—we're less apt to be hijacked by a disowned part. The way we can call our exiled parts home is by cultivating self-compassion or a peaceful presence toward them. While it may sound like fluff, there's hard science to back its transformative power.[54] Beyond boosting resilience, emotional stability, and mood,[55] self-compassion can also improve your relationship.

In a study on the role of self-compassion in romantic relationships, Kristin Neff and Natasha Beretvas found that individuals high in self-compassion tend to display warmth and affection for their partners. They are tolerant of their own and their partner's flaws, accept responsibility for misdeeds, and are less defensive in conflicts. In contrast, those low in self-compassion are more controlling and verbally aggressive. They score higher on measures for depression, anxiety, and neurotic perfectionism.[56]

Further studies suggest that individuals who score high on self-compassion experience more relational satisfaction and a greater willingness to compromise.[57] However, it is important not to mistake self-compassion for its competitive cousin, self-esteem, which rises and falls based on how we rank ourselves against others.[58] In our striving for high self-esteem, we often pump ourselves up by putting others down.[59] In relationships, this can lead to battles about who's right and wrong. Moreover, high self-esteem is a weak predictor of relationship satisfaction and caring behaviors. It can foster jealousy, anger, and aggression, qualities that undermine erotic cooperation.[60]

There are no winners or losers on the naked path. However, if our self-esteem is dependent on feeling competent as a lover, we will resist hearing feedback. We are likely to be critical of ourselves and our partner when we have a disappointing or imperfect sexual experience. In contrast, self-compassion helps us accept sexual variability as a feature of real-life sex. It also fosters a sense of interconnectedness, which may be why researchers have found indications that self-compassion can promote secure attachment.[61] One self-compassion practice involves sending the warm rays of the sun to different parts of us and then to all beings that suffer. We might repeat the words:

May you be happy
May you be free of suffering
May you know peace.

Self-compassion is a way to meet our needs for comfort, kindness, and belonging. We give ourselves love and acceptance when our partner is unable to provide these. We are not trying to bolster our self-esteem or validate our experience. We are not giving ourselves a pep talk; or telling ourselves to buck up and "get over it." Instead, we are "being with" our suffering by practicing peaceful presence.[62]

We might imagine that we are a compassionate grown-up meeting our younger self, possibly letting the little one cry it out. We can use Cupid's wings to wrap ourselves in kindness when we feel sad and alone. In an ideal world, those wings would come from another human, especially when we are little. If this was the case for you, you are likely to reach for others when you hurt. You trust that arms will be waiting. Some of us, though, got far too little wrapping, or none at all. This deficit can mean that even when we want comfort, we push it away.

In our RIL or vicious cycle, we have no choice but to wrap ourselves. Our partners need their wings to stay airborne or to wrap themselves. When we practice peaceful presence, we acknowledge that the pain we feel is real and also very human. We use our pain to foster a sense of connection to the vast web of humanity by remembering that from the beginning of time, many others have felt just this way.

## THE CARE CYCLE AND CREATING OUR LOVING CONTAINER

### The Three Rs: Reveal, Reach, and Repair

When our commitment to knowing and revealing ourselves is greater than the need to hide, protect, or defend—or to blame

others—we pull on a thread that promises to unravel all the layers of protection that keep us isolated and disconnected.
—Jett Psaris and Marlena S. Lyons[63]

I recommend a set of practices that I call the "three Rs," as part of the care cycle (see figure 3.5, "The Care Cycle"). While the PREP process is a way to work with yourself to interrupt the vicious cycle, the three Rs are an investment in your relationship. They are how we love *actively*. If you practice regularly, the three Rs will strengthen your relational container and cultivate a spirit of cooperation that you can both use to hold the hard stuff together.

### R1: REVEAL

Love takes off masks that we fear we cannot live without and know we cannot live within.
—James Baldwin[64]

When Max and Eric reconnect after completing the PREP process, Eric says that he now realizes that he is acting superior because underneath he feels rejected and alone. This disclosure invites a softening in Max who reveals that old feelings of being "stupid" were underneath his dismissive behavior toward Eric. In a quid pro quo relationship, the governing stance is "I'll show you mine, if you'll show me yours." At stage 3, our nakedness is unconditional. We reveal our vulnerability because we choose intimacy over protection.

It takes courage to share our soft underbelly with our partners, but when we do so by exposing our hurts and fears, we also become allies on this curious and adventurous path. When we're in our reciprocal interaction loop, we hide our vulnerability by acting opposite to how we feel. We appear powerful when we feel weak. We act superior when we feel inadequate. We have to learn to let each other know "what is going on behind the scenes," says Welwood.[65] It is the only way to break the habit of letting our protective states rule us.

Many of our protective strategies are automatic; they arise in less than one twenty-fifth of a second.[66] We yell instead of asking for help.

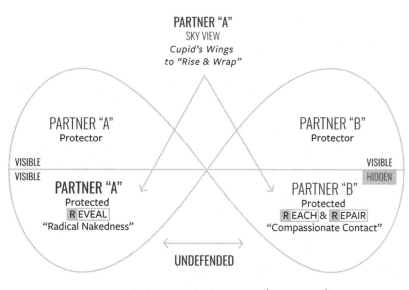

## FIGURE 3.5 THE CARE CYCLE (THE 3 RS)

The Care Cycle consists of the three Rs, which are how we love actively. Here partner A is initiating the cycle by **revealing** their discoveries from mindful self-study to partner B. Partner A can also **reach** into partner B's "underneath" and compassionately guess B's hidden pain. Partner A may initiate a process to **repair** the hurt they may have caused partner B when partner A was acting from their protector.

When our partner shouts back, we feel more helpless and alone, and the world seems without mercy. We don't realize that if we merely say, "I'm afraid you'll reject me if I show my full aliveness," or, "I'd like to try that role-play, but I'm afraid of looking silly," that we invite care rather than conflict.

I call revealing the underneath "radical nakedness." It is naked because it is undefended. It is radical because we show what we most want to hide. While removing our armor sounds like giving up—or worse still, weakness—to our protector, it is by no means a "weak" position. We have the most power to change the loop from here. Telling the naked truth is a disarming move, and it invites a like response from our partner. It helps you as a couple break the cycle of relating to each other's protective strategies, which is essential if we want to access our PEP.

## R2: REACH

Radical nakedness is the first *R* of the care cycle. The second *R* is to *reach* into our partner's underneath. It helps to remember that your partner's protector is just a front for a hidden part that feels unlovable, alone, helpless, or afraid. To make the reach we ask ourselves, "What is underneath our partner's intensity, harshness, sarcasm, or withdrawal?" "Is our partner feeling sad, powerless, incompetent, terrified, or rejected?" To answer this question, we draw on our knowledge of our partner's core wounds and try to guess what is causing the pain.

Once we have a guess, we can tell our partner what we seem to understand about their experience. It doesn't matter if we are right; it is the intention to bring empathy to our partner that opens *our* hearts— and possibly theirs. A simple statement is enough, such as: "I wonder if you feel lost and unlovable right now." Or, "I imagine you feel worthless when I talk to you this way." Or, "I'm guessing that your domineering dictator is keeping you from feeling humiliated."

We call reaching for our partner's underneath "compassionate contact" because we are "feeling with" our partner. Our heart has to be open to be able to do this. If we are telling our partner what we know—from on high—then the contact won't work. Sounding righteous or superior will only evoke more of our partner's protector.

Compassionate contact is how we stay awake to the fact that we are not the only vulnerable one. Our partner is having an experience of equal measure to our own. "When caught up in an impasse," Sheinkman and Fishbane tell us, "partners don't see the hurt, but only the self-protective shield of the other."[67] At stage 3, we hold the aspiration to have this empathic understanding of the other person and to love them—even when our needs are not immediately satisfied.[68]

## R3: REPAIRING RUPTURES

When first in love, you and your partner are in synch much of the time. Eventually, however, you're tired, and your partner wants to go for a long walk. You want sex, and your partner wants to stay up and work. While the cultural narrative is that love relationships are smooth and easy, all relationships, including those between caregivers and their children, are fraught with mismatched or uncoordinated exchanges.

Remarkably, out of 15,536,000 second-by-second exchanges between an adult and an awake infant in the first year of life, only 30 percent are attuned, according to the Harvard researcher Ed Tronic.[69] Here, attuned means that the adult and child are in synchronized states. For the adult, it also means they are receiving and accurately interpreting signals from the child. On the contrary, the data suggest that instead of being in synch, more often than not, caregivers miss or misinterpret their infant's cues.

In adult relationships, a rupture may also result from missed signals or by being in different states. Sometimes, these misses result in hurt feelings. Perhaps you gave feedback to your partner about the kind of touch that you'd like, and instead of welcoming your coaching, your partner got defensive. Now, neither of you are in the mood for sex, nor do you feel very close.

In parent-child relationships, it is the bigger, more mature person's job to repair ruptures. Even as adults, we need our bigger self to be online to come back into a loving connection. At stage 3, we attend to our states and use the PREP process precisely for this reason.

Sometimes, it is possible to quickly repair the rupture and move from mismatched to matching states. Such a repair process can happen verbally or nonverbally. We may take time to hold each other or issue a simple apology. On other occasions, we have to go further. It is easy to imagine that a protector part was mean-spirited if we were in our "vicious cycle." In such instances, our repair process involves hearing the impact we have had, showing remorse, and seeing what kind of mending is necessary to right things again.

Uncoupling intention from impact is imperative in repair processes. If I step on your toe, it hurts, even if I didn't mean to cause harm. I need to own that. On the other hand, many of us are walking around with a broken toe, which means we are vulnerable to reinjury.[70] Fred Luskin of the Stanford Forgiveness Center claims that the person who carries old wounds should also apologize for their reactivity.[71] A mindful approach is "both/and," which in this case, involves *both* repairing the present-time relational breach *and* exploring the longer-standing wound.

## From Adversaries to Allies: The Skill of Mindful Coinvestigation

After Max and Eric become aware of their protector and protected parts, my next task is to teach them how to use mindful coinvestigation to explore their sexual relationship. Since Max complained about Eric's "constant" appeals for sex, I suggest we start by exploring Max's side of the equation. I check for consent, and they agree.

Max has softened considerably from the activity of diagramming their RIL. He concedes that for a long time the "cock grab" had been exciting, even relieving. Now it merely irritates Max, although he doesn't know why. I ask Max if he is curious about his irritation. He replies, "The gesture is so crude." I propose that instead of talking about it, we do mindful coinvestigation. This technique turns something aversive into a little research project that is done together as a team.

Being a person of action, Eric immediately takes to the notion of an experiment. I tell him that he will have to go slow, though; otherwise, Max's protectors will take over again, and Max won't be able to stay curious. Eric nods, indicating understanding. For the experiment, I suggest that Eric slowly move his hand towards Max's crotch while Max studies anything that changes in his inner world. I instruct Eric to pause anytime Max puts his hand up to signal he is noticing something.

As preparation, we spend a minute in mindful meditation. I invite Max to summon his curiosity and "inner observer" before we begin. He closes his eyes and moves awareness into the present moment with the help of his breathing. The purpose of first becoming mindful is to slow down enough to come off of automatic pilot. Being in a mindful state means we are able to notice subtle changes in our experience that are missed when we are fast and reactive.

I then instruct Max to open his eyes when he is ready, and Eric very slowly reaches for Max's crotch. Almost immediately, Max's hand goes up. I ask what is happening. Max says he feels angry. "How do you know?" I ask. "What exactly is happening inside of you?" Max describes something that feels like "hot red steel" in the middle of his throat. I encourage him to stay with it, but he signals for Eric to resume. Right away, Max makes the pause signal again. This time, Max says he feels something in his hands. As he stays with his hands, he feels the impulse to swat Eric's hand away.

I tell Max to let the impulse in his hand happen in slow motion, and they hesitantly start a game of "push hands." They both seem very engaged. After a while, Max has trouble concealing a smile. "It's kind of fun, huh?" I remark. Max smiles broadly now and says he enjoys having the power to stop Eric with his hands. I encourage Max to stay with his enjoyment, which has spread into his face and belly. After a good while, Max realizes that the overt sexual proposition is too fast for him. He wants to follow his course instead of always taking Eric's lead.

I encourage Max to be with this sense of wanting to follow his course and wonder if he remembers a time, possibly in his early life, when that wasn't possible. Max has only a vague glimmer of being dominated in some way a long time back. He senses giving in to other people's wishes and now feels angry about it. Max realizes he has been "going along" with Eric for most of their relationship. His aversive reaction to the cock grab threads to a previously unacknowledged feeling of powerlessness.

In a session the following day, Eric explores his part of the dynamic. Eric wonders why he needs to have sex to feel okay about himself. He admits that he starts to feel anxious when too much time goes by without it. Exploring the anxiety is a good starting point for an experiment. I ask Eric what Max does when he says no to sex. Eric thinks for a minute then laughs as he says, "It's like he swats me away." Eric makes the gesture. I ask Eric if he wants to do some mindful coinvestigation using this motion as a trigger. He agrees.

Eric closes his eyes and gets mindful. I tell Eric to open his eyes when he is ready to receive the trigger. Once he does so, Max makes a swatting gesture with his right hand. Eric realizes that Max needs to add a couple of things to make the triggering gesture just right. First, he has to drop his head back when he swats. Second, Max has to roll his eyes in an expression of disgust. Since Max doesn't know that he does this, Eric shows him the move.

After practicing a couple of times, we start over. Eric gets mindful and closes his eyes. When he opens them, Max makes the agreed upon gesture. Eric notices some hardness move across his upper body, like a shield. I also note that he is gritting his teeth. I invite Eric to stay with this shielding and exaggerate it by 10 percent. Eric tightens and releases a few times. Then, I ask what his body seems to be saying when it mobilizes this way. He pauses to study the shielding and then answers, "I'm not going to feel this." "Oh, so the shield is helping you not feel something," I acknowledge, adding, "Maybe sense that for a bit longer."

After another minute, I ask Eric if he wants to experiment with letting the shield down by 10 percent to see what he might feel. Eric starts to do that and very quickly reassembles the protection. "Seems like you got a whiff of something you don't like," I say. I also detect a slight tremor in Eric's body. He seems to be searching for something and scrunches his face. "I just had a flash of my parents in front of their Cadillac Eldorado," he reports. He studies the image some more and realizes that his parents are dropping him off at boarding school. Eric is back in his memory now. He doesn't want to go to this school but is trying hard not to feel how scared and alone he feels. The shield seems to help.

The young Eric feels like he is being "shipped off." Eric now remembers that as a child, he felt like he was a nuisance to his parents. Eric's sadness is evident now, and Max's eyes water too. Eric realizes that he hates needing anything from Max but that the old feeling of being a nuisance comes up when Max "swats" him away. He also realizes that he has been using sex to reassure himself that someone wants him. Now, Eric can't hold back his tears. He starts to sob, big sobs for the boy who felt like a nuisance. Max is kissing his hand. "I want you," Max says.

When the wave of emotion passes, Eric looks up at Max and apologizes. He can see that his insistence on having sex was to reassure himself that he was wanted. As Eric is speaking, it's clear that his armor is not there. He is completely naked. Max's heart opens as Max sees Eric's vulnerability. Although Eric is making the repair, it is Max who now feels terrible for reinjuring this boy. Now that Eric and Max know about each other's underlying wounds, they look for ways to help Max feel empowered, while helping Eric to feel wanted.

Eric and Max are ready to approach each other as an erotic team. For starters, Eric asks Max how he can express his interest in sex in a more inclusive way moving forward. An image appears in Max's mind. He turns Eric's hands face up, and stretches Eric's left arm out like a host might signal "After you," or "Right this way." I ask Max for the words that go with the gesture. He pauses and answers, "Shall we dance?"

The couple is actively practicing the art of erotic cooperation. Max and Eric agree to view their next erotic encounter as a dance, with both taking turns leading and following. They decide to pause and check in with each other every few minutes to see if Max is still in harmony with his course. Eric agrees to stop and share if his old fears of being unwanted surface. They leave feeling openhearted and united in forging a new and more naked path.

"Being deeply loved by someone gives you strength while loving someone deeply gives you courage," says Lao Tzu.[72] Erotic cooperation involves building a relational container in which you can meet the challenges of life, and real-life sex, with clasped hands. Sexual difficulties can bring you closer together if you get naked with one another. When partners understand the wounds carried by each other, hearts open, doors unlock, and protectors don't have to work so hard.

## MINDFUL ACTIVITIES AND NAKED REFLECTIONS

. . . . . . . . . . . . . . . . . . . . . . . . . . . . . . . . . . . . . . . . . . . . . . . . . . . . . . . . . . . . . . . . . . .

### Getting to Know Your Protector and Protected Parts

. . . . . . . . . . . . . . . . . . . . . . . . . . . . . . . . . . . . . . . . . . . . . . . . . . . . . . . . . . . . . . . . . . .

Before you begin, choose a specific conflict that you can remember well and refer to throughout the exercise. Ideally, it will be related to sex, but it doesn't have to be. Our protector and protected parts show up in all conflict situations where we rely on protective strategies. For this exercise, you can use figure 3.6 as a worksheet or reproduce the image on a sheet of paper.

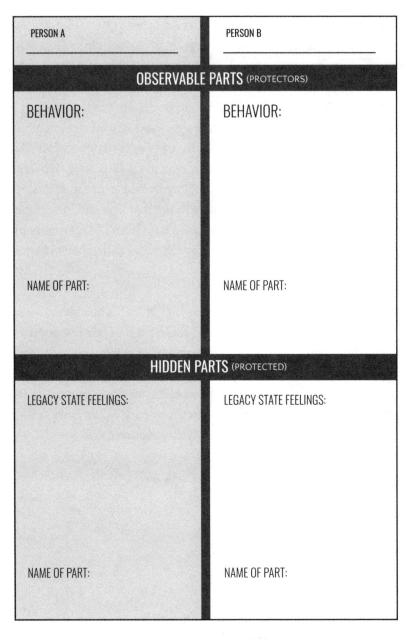

PERSON A _____

PERSON B _____

**OBSERVABLE PARTS** (PROTECTORS)

BEHAVIOR:

BEHAVIOR:

NAME OF PART:

NAME OF PART:

**HIDDEN PARTS** (PROTECTED)

LEGACY STATE FEELINGS:

LEGACY STATE FEELINGS:

NAME OF PART:

NAME OF PART:

FIGURE 3.6 GETTING TO KNOW YOUR PROTECTOR
AND PROTECTED PARTS

—from Halko Weiss

Use this worksheet to complete the activity, or reproduce the image on a piece of paper.

## Step 1: Complete the Upper-Right Portion of the RIL Diagram

### Getting to Know Partner B's Protector

To begin this exercise, choose who will go first. Partner A is going to imagine they are back in the conflict situation. List the behaviors you see in partner B during the conflict. As you do this, avoid making interpretations. For instance, instead of describing partner B's behavior as "arrogant," "intimidating," or "manipulative," translate those interpretations into things you can observe. What is your partner doing with their face, their posture, their movements, their energy, and their gestures? What key phrases do they use? Be detailed and objective. List eight to ten observations in the upper-right portion of the RIL diagram.

If you are doing this exercise together, partner B can be your scribe. Keep listing behavioral observations until you feel that there's nothing more to add to the list. You can also go to pages 68–69 for examples of what you might be observing in your partner.

It's okay to laugh during this activity (or cry or feel any other emotion). At the same time, it also helps to be in your observing self more than your experiencing self.

Once you have finished the list, try to come up with a name for your partner's protector. If you are doing this exercise together, ask partner B if they have a name for their protector. You can both brainstorm names, using literary characters, villains from action movies, animals, or anything else that captures the archetypal force of this protector (e.g., the "Grim Avenger," the "Refrigerator," the "Know-it-all," or the "Lunging Tiger.") If your partner feels hurt or disagrees, find a name that works for the both of you.

## Step 2: Complete the Upper-Left Portion of the RIL Diagram

### Getting to Know Partner A's Protector

Switch roles so that partner B lists partner A's behaviors during the conflict. Partner A can be the scribe. When you have completed the list, choose a name for partner A's protector.

## Step 3: Complete Partner B's Bottom Quadrant

### Getting to Know Partner B's Protected Part

To feel what lies underneath this protective dynamic, partner B will first become mindful. Slow down, then pause to feel into yourself, becoming aware of your body. Become sensitive to tiny shifts in your experience as you breathe, and notice the effects of the exercise so far.

You will be using mental imagery to trigger your legacy state. Imagine you are back in the conflict situation right now. Make this as real as possible in your felt experience. Observe partner A's behavior during the conflict (the actions of the protector that you listed above). What happens in you now in response to those behaviors?

Turn your awareness from imagining partner A's behavior to noticing yourself. What kind of state starts to form in you? What feelings begin to emerge? You are going for vulnerable emotions like fear, confusion, sadness, and worthlessness. If feelings like anger come up or impulses, such as withdrawing, see what those things are protecting you from experiencing.

What deeper distress is underneath?

What would happen if they were not there?

What would be exposed?

What kind of pain and vulnerability would you otherwise experience without their help?

Give yourself plenty of time for this step.

Share these things with your partner as you become aware of them. Partner A can be the scribe.

### Naming the Protected Part

As you sense into your legacy state, what might you call this part? What name might capture the essence of this part of you and its experience? Again, you can draw from myths and fairy tales, animals, or characters in movies to come up with a name for this part (e.g., Orphan Annie, Lost Puppy, Ugly Duckling, E.T.)

## Appreciating Your Protector

You can start to understand that protectors are truly protecting you from feeling this. As you feel into the old feelings, you or your partner can ask how far this collection of emotions, body sensations, and beliefs goes back in time. What does it remind you of from your early life? Afterward, be tender with yourself.

## Step 4: Complete Partner A's Bottom Quadrant

### Getting to Know Partner A's Protected Part

Switch roles. Now it is partner A's turn to identity a legacy state. Repeat the steps from above. If you are diagramming alone, you will have to fill in your partner's protected legacy state. The hardest step is to imagine the impact your protector has on your partner. Try to put yourself in your partner's shoes, feel underneath the bluster and sense into their vulnerable legacy state.

Afterward, take time to explore the reciprocity of your dynamic. Notice how when partner A's legacy state is evoked—without being aware of it—that their protector immediately and automatically tries to help. How does partner A's protector evoke partner B's legacy state? Notice how partner B's protector works to help partner B from feeling their own legacy state. Sense how this interaction could go on infinitely unless someone does something different.

When you start seeing this dynamic is a system made up of each partner's protector and protected parts, you are already less identified with it. Having space around this tight knot helps it start to loosen, allowing you to feel compassion for each other. As we disidentify, which means observing the pattern rather than reacting from inside of it, we are jumping out of the system. Disidentification is the first step in interrupting the loop before it goes too far.

As you become more familiar with the RIL, you can diagram it in your head, pausing to feel what lies underneath in real time. Alternatively, you can take a mindful pause during conflicts and journey down to what is lying underneath to see what you are protecting. Be sure to reveal your discoveries. Remember, revealing what your protector is protecting (i.e., being radically naked) is the power position. You are interrupting the loop to move back into an undefended exchange.

## Variation: Mindful Coinvestigation

If you are doing this activity with your partner, coach them to take on the posture or facial expression of their protector. Note: It does not have to be what they do in real life; instead, it is a representation of how they appear to you when you are in the loop. You can then explore what lies underneath in real time, as you sense what begins to happen inside of you and how your protector wants to help you manage the experience.

## Naked Reflections

What did you discover about yourself that was surprising
and new?
What did you discover about your partner that was surprising
and new?
What can you do to interrupt the cycle when you are stuck in
your loop?
How can you practice PREP when you need to?
How can you use the three Rs to transform your stuck cycle
into a cycle of care?

# 4.

# EROTIC TRANSFORMATION

## Healing and Growing through Sex

If you can find a path with no obstacles, it probably
doesn't lead anywhere.
—FRANK A. CLARK[1]

Kyle, an attractive man in his late fifties, has felt sexually insecure for
most of his life. Dressed in red high-tops and loose-fitting jeans, he
shifts uneasily in the overstuffed chair. Looking downcast, Kyle tells me
that in his twenties and thirties, he was a "terrible" lover. When performance anxiety got the better of him, he would lose his erection or come
too soon. Those situations were so shameful that Kyle "fled the scene"
afterward to avoid exposing his feelings of inadequacy.

By his account, it was something of a miracle that Kyle met Sienna
when he was thirty-nine. As a teenager, Kyle's secret fantasy was to
be initiated into the mysteries of sex by an experienced older woman.
Some twenty years later, Sienna certainly fit the bill. She was a compassionate and assured forty-five-year-old who also loved sex. Moreover,
the chemistry between them was so intimate and trusting that Kyle's
worries seemed to vanish miraculously. For the first time in his life, Kyle
felt like a competent lover.

That feeling lasted for the first six years of their marriage. Then,
without warning, Kyle's anxiety returned with a vengeance. Small

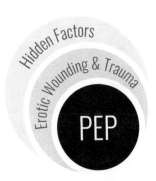

FIGURE 4.1 CHAPTER 4 PEP BARRIERS

mishaps before or during sex would rattle Kyle, causing his erection to wane. Consequently, worries about performance are preoccupying him again. In our session, Kyle wonders, "What is the source of my anxiety? Why is it back? Can it change, or am I destined to feel like a sexual failure for the rest of my life?"

Kyle is, understandably, disheartened, but he's asking the right questions. Why, after so many years of empowering sexual experiences, is Kyle avoiding sex with his wife? What is behind his anxiety, and can he break free of lifelong patterns that leave him feeling sexually inadequate, dissatisfied, and stuck?

## THE HIDDEN FACTORS: OUR PEP-LIMITING IMPRINTS

If you are like most couples, then you or your partner has struggled with complex emotions and preoccupations that have taken the joy out of sex. When this is the case, we can suspect that imprints are at work. Many of our unpleasant or downright triggering reactions to sex are due to sex-negative messages that have been imprinted unconsciously, as well as wounds from childhood that get transferred to sex. As a result, we lose confidence in ourselves or become troubled by our sexual feelings and behaviors.

All of our experiences, including any wounding or trauma, sexual or not, goes into our "imprint portfolio." Some imprints cast a pall over our erotic life and form an invisible barrier to experiencing our pure erotic potential. It is because they are invisible that I refer to these imprints as the "hidden factors." So, while billed as a fun, pleasurable, and connecting activity, sex also has a darker side. Even in—and indeed *because of*—the trust and love in a safe, committed relationship, our lovemaking can stir up unpleasant emotions and body sensations.

In the West, we mostly try to solve problems or avoid them. We may seek "happy endings" through sex while shunning the complicated emotions that arise when we get triggered. While avoiding sex may seem preferable to feeling anxious and ashamed, when we erect barriers between ourselves and our pain, our issues don't move. For this reason, avoidance can lead to what is called arrested development. However, when we approach our hidden factors mindfully, and especially as a team, we can find a portal to healing and transformation.

## Five Features of the Hidden Factors

To start our healing, we need to be able to recognize the five main features of the hidden factors. It is also crucial to know why "trying to figure it out" only takes us so far:

1. We get potent sexual education lessons from our earliest imprints, or memories-as-learning, that are "known but unremembered."[2]

2. These experiences, along with the family, religious, and cultural messages we encode, become the basis of internal models and beliefs that shape our erotic lives, outside of awareness.[3]

3. We can think of our hidden factors as emotional and bodily tattoos—durable but invisible at first because of the arousal surge at stage 1.

4. Our hidden factors remain invisible until stage 2 when they start to generate unpleasant reactions, confusion, and sometimes avoidance of sex.

5. They are triggered by—but also illuminated by—the "black light syndrome," which in scientific circles is called state-dependent memory.[4]

## 1. IMPRINT PORTFOLIOS: OUR SEX ED THAT IS UNREMEMBERED BUT NOT FORGOTTEN

Way before the "birds and the bees" talk (if there ever was one), you were observing how your caregivers wore their sexuality, whether openly in bold, colorful designs or "buttoned up" in muted textures and hues. You were sensing the feeling tone when conversations featured sex, even though you were probably too young to fully understand them.

As with everything we learn, our sexual education is not merely a verbal discourse; it is also an emotional exchange.[5] We are resonating with the *state* of the messenger as conveyed by their facial expression, posture, and voice tone. These experiences encode in the deeper structures of our brains outside of conscious awareness, which means they are difficult—if not impossible—to recall.[6] Moreover, the takeaway of this early emotional learning lasts longer than words ever will.[7]

## 2. INTERNAL MODELS AND LIMITING BELIEFS: THE INVISIBLE SHAPERS OF OUR EROTIC LIFE

Our own experiences—along with cultural, group, and familial imprints—form internal models (sometimes called "core beliefs" or "schemas") in our psyches, shaping our perceptions without us recognizing their organizing power.[8] For example, we may think oral sex is okay but feel disgusted when we have it.

Without words, by eighteen months of age, we have already established internal models that pertain to how others will treat us and how we have to be to survive in the world.[9] Our models inform our general beliefs for the lives we anticipate as well as our attitudes toward sex. Additionally, in whatever way we identify—ethnically, racially, culturally, and sexually—we all imprint our subgroups' models of healthy, appropriate, and "hot" sex, as well as perverse and "wrong" sex. Most likely, you have models that prevent you from expressing yourself sexually as fully as you desire.

Some limiting beliefs are specifically about sex. They can show up as, "Sex is dirty or dangerous," or "I'm bad for enjoying pleasure." If this is the case, we will hide or exile our desires or feel guilty if we "indulge." Quite often, our unconscious models about sex are knotted with more general models about self and others in PEP-defying ways.

For example, if my model is that I'll be hurt if I open up, I may lose my desire for anyone I love. If I carry a model that "I'm not safe," I won't be able to relax into pleasure. If I "know" I can't shape things to my liking, I will hold back on expressing my preferences. I will wait for my partner to initiate, even though doing so may curb my enthusiasm for sex, as was undoubtedly the case for Max.

When we identify with beliefs like these, our perceptual filters blind us to experiences to the contrary. We automatically scan for evidence that supports our most ingrained views, and naturally, we find it.[10] Nonetheless, it's important to remember that the power behind our hidden factors is that they shape our feelings and behaviors outside of awareness.[11] For example, Max didn't have a specific memory; only a felt sense that he had to go along with others rather than following his course. So, while Eric's leadership in pursuing sex seemed to confirm this belief, Eric's behavior was not motivated by a desire to overpower Max. It was to help Eric feel wanted.

## 3. EMOTIONAL AND SOMATIC TATTOOS: INVISIBLE BUT POISONOUS

Everything we know and remember—indeed, everything we are, our beliefs and values and personalities and character—is encoded in the connections that neurons make in our brains.
—Sharon Begley[12]

The extent to which the coupling of our neurons affects us is truly epic. Early sensory and emotional imprints shape our thoughts, psyches, bodies, and sexuality without us knowing when or how they have taken root.[13] They are like emotional and somatic tattoos, made without our knowledge or consent in poisonous, phosphorescent ink. These tattoos cover our bodies a little or a lot, but we all have them.

Just as implicit rules of grammar shape our speech, our implicit learning determines how we make love, whether or not we issue or accept advances, and what we find aversive and arousing.[14] Moreover, our initial associations between one thing and another—such as sex and shame—are the most enduring. Once experience goes into long-term storage, it wants to stay in there for keeps, even in conditions of dementia.[15]

Our hidden factors can make us feel marked because they are so hard to remove. Fortunately, research shows that we can decouple the neural pathways that are causing us problems so that our hidden factors no longer run us sexually. Moreover, your partner can help you detoxify your poisonous tattoos, so they become a symbol of resilience rather than a source of pain and stigma.

### 4. OUT OF SIGHT: STATE-DEPENDENT AND AUTOMATIC

We usually can't recall the experiences filed in our emotional memory because they encode outside of awareness.[16] However, certain sensations, smells, words, and activities during sex act as cues that trigger our hidden factors.[17] Then, everything we've learned about sex—implicitly—rushes forward, often as a body memory when we are making love. We may not know what's happening, only that we suddenly feel triggered.[18]

To understand why this happens, we need to know a bit about how we make and retrieve memories. One explanation is that our brain functions as a camera and makes photographs of our experiences by firing a sequence of neurons.[19] When this same sequence fires repeatedly, these neurons wire together, which is how experience moves from its temporary holding facility into long-term storage. Of course, sometimes we experience something so traumatic that one exposure is enough to lay down the memory.

Memories are "retrieved" when the same sequence of neurons fire again, which is most likely to happen when we are in a similar feeling state to when we took the "photograph."[20] This means that what we have learned about sex is more likely to be retrieved when we are in a sexual state.

## 5. THE BAD NEWS AND GOOD NEWS: STAGE 2 AND THE BLACK LIGHT SYNDROME

A strange and often confusing hallmark of the hidden factors is that they emerge well after the first blush of romance settles into a secure attachment. We may wonder why we were able to enjoy a vibrant and satisfying sex life before, without getting triggered. It is because the passion cocktail I described in chapter 1 creates a temporary arousal spike that overrides our PEP-limiting imprints. It's as if our imprint portfolio goes into "cold" storage for a while. In Kyle's case, "a while" was six years; but for some people, it may be merely six months.

Like a black light revealing a previously hidden image, our bodily and emotional tattoos become ever more visible at stage 2. Now our imprint portfolio opens during sex, automatically, and eros illuminates the insecurities and wounds hidden in safe storage in our non-sexual states. For this reason, we may find that our body says, "No!" to the suggestion of sex, even though we want to connect to our partner. Or we end up feeling upset, fearful, embarrassed, or exposed when we make love. Black light syndrome can feel raw and revealing, weighing down on the relationship until these newly illuminated scars are dealt with in the light of mindful awareness.

Many sexual enrichment programs avoid these complex emotional reactions, but no romantic gesture or seduction technique will enroll the part of you that is unconsciously ambivalent about sex. Likewise, until you address your hidden factors, learning ways to have mind-blowing orgasms will be useless because you either won't apply them or will lose any short-term gains over time.

When the hidden factors light up, our reactions are fast and automatic. We may go from turned on to flatlined, ecstatic to guilt-ridden in a matter of seconds without knowing why. The reason for our state change is that during sex, "sparks fly" in a near-literal sense. A network of neurons fire in concert, creating a symphony of feelings, images, thoughts, and sensations that either boost or trounce our PEP.

At first glance, this seems to be only bad news. Sex becomes complicated—and naked—at stage 2. However, we also get to see the well-formed beliefs and patterns we hold, which affect our experience of sex and ourselves as a sexual being. That is the "good news/bad news" about a long-term, sexual relationship. It is for this reason that committed sex is very naked, and at the same time, full of healing potential.

## HOW CAN WE HEAL AND GROW THROUGH SEX?

By embracing the both/and approach, of using sex for *both* pleasure *and* healing, you can transform your hidden factors. Stage 3 couples wake up together by working through erotic issues as a mindful team. They practice mindful self-study and mindful coinvestigation, skills that allow them to work with their PEP-limiting imprints and explore their triggers separately and together.

They also consciously cultivate something called *response-agility*,[21] wherein they fluidly shift back and forth between making love to exploring barriers that emerge during an encounter. Thus, rather than viewing their presence as a disruptor, stage 3 couples welcome the appearance of the hidden factors as an opportunity to heal old imprints and shame marks.

## SOMATIC SELF-ATTUNEMENT: A KEY TO HEALING AND GROWTH

The body is essential to accessing and transforming the hidden factors. As we encode much of our early learning in the body,[22] working with our "felt sense" is how we gain access to our implicit memory system.[23] As we saw with Eric, we can mindfully direct our attention to a body reaction, such as tightness in the chest, and let emotions, images, and memories come into awareness. When meaning emerges through the body, we are engaging in what neuroscientists call "bottom-up processing."[24] This approach works better than trying to "figure it out" cognitively.[25]

## Triggered Again! Now What?

The cure for pain is in the pain.

—Rumi[26]

On the road to our PEP, Cupid's leaden arrow may puncture our tire. These emotional blowouts are in response to one or more "triggers." As mentioned, a smell, visual image, voice tone, or sensation can evoke an unpleasant emotional or physical reaction or series of responses that "go off" when we are having sex. These responses are often associated with our early emotional learning.

In the moment, when vestiges of the past intrude on the present, they can turn a loving and pleasurable encounter into a painful reenactment of a wounding experience from the past. For this reason, you will want to greet these sexual relics with a curious and gentle heart, even though your impulse may be to withdraw or blame your partner.

Reflecting on his youth, Kyle admits that he always felt deeply conflicted about his sexuality. His father was an underemployed alcoholic who was violent on occasion. As an only child, Kyle felt protective of his mother, who leaned on Kyle and also expected Kyle to be a different kind of man.

During the women's movement of the late 1970s, Kyle's fear of his sexuality intensified when he absorbed messages that men were insensitive brutes. Consequently, Kyle found it impossible to believe that the women he was having sex with were enjoying it. For this reason, he tried to get through the act of intercourse as quickly as possible. Because sex had been for release rather than exploration, Kyle never learned what women want.

The effects of this backstory only became conscious to Kyle after a few sessions of mindful self-study. Before that, he felt disconnected and vulnerable during sex, blaming himself or Sienna when he felt triggered. I call this pattern of defense the "defend cycle" (see figure 4.2).

In today's session, Kyle wants to understand why he reacts so strongly to a facial expression that Sienna makes when she appears

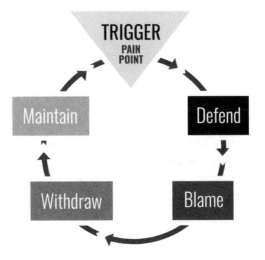

**FIGURE 4.2 DEFEND CYCLE**

In the defend cycle, we rely on protective strategies to avoid experiencing pain. In so doing, we maintain rather than grow both ourselves and our PEP.

to be unhappy with him. Kyle reports that when he sees that look on her face, he immediately gets angry and shuts down sexually. He and Sienna are committed to undertaking this research as a team and agree to explore the trigger using mindful coinvestigation. I call this practice of researching triggers using mindful self-study or coinvestigation the "befriend cycle" (see figure 4.3).

First, Kyle coaches Sienna to pinch her face and furrow her brow in a particular way so he can study his aversive reaction. She tries it, and he does some tweaking until he feels a clench in his stomach, and says, "Yes, exactly!" Next, Kyle closes his eyes and becomes mindful. He is entering an open, receptive state in which he can observe subtle changes in his inner world. At his signal, I instruct Sienna to make the expression again, and for Kyle to open his eyes. He looks at Sienna for about three seconds then closes his eyes to study his reaction to the trigger.

Kyle feels the clench in his belly again. I direct him to stay with it in a curious, open way. After a minute or so of opening and closing his eyes, Kyle reports that there's something familiar in Sienna's face, something that reminds him of his mother. He feels a tightening across his ribs and a "sucking in" feeling in his lower belly when he says this. I invite Kyle

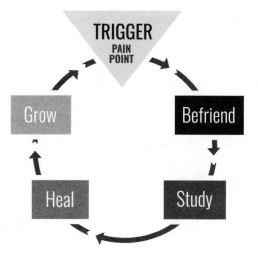

FIGURE 4.3 BEFRIEND CYCLE

In the befriend cycle, we research triggers and pain points using the skills of mindful self-study and coinvestigation to support healing and growth.

to stay with the sensations and to study them precisely. As we saw with Eric previously, when we are mindful, our body sensations can link us to other times we have felt like this.

Kyle flashes on a memory of an unpleasant exchange with his mother when he was thirteen. I talk to Kyle in the present tense and ask what is happening between them. Kyle says his mother seems to want him to know that his father does "disgusting" things. She doesn't elaborate, but it's clear the "disgusting" things are sexual. She is pinching her face and furrowing her brows as she is speaking. Kyle is surprised, and expresses bitter amusement, to make this connection. He can see that Sienna's face sometimes looks the same way to him.

I ask Kyle to notice what is happening inside of him now. Kyle is wondering if his mother is expressing disapproval of him without saying so. The young Kyle is starting to feel anxious and ashamed. Kyle tells me that he doesn't want to be anything like his father, but he is also quite fascinated by sex. After acknowledging his feelings, I ask Kyle what his impulse is as he senses into this bind. He considers this for a while and answers, "I am trying to hide my interest in sex, so I don't repel my mother."

A look of surprised recognition comes across Kyle's face like he sees something about himself in a new way. I ask Kyle how he is doing this hiding. Again, Kyle pauses to explore his felt sense. Eventually, he says, "I am sucking in my belly and tightening my ribs." Kyle immediately sees the link between his feelings of shame and his efforts to disconnect from his sexuality. He now also understands why Sienna's look of disapproval is so triggering. It evokes strong feelings of guilt, which he pushes away by extinguishing his sexual feelings altogether.

Kyle looks sad and a little withered in his body. Observing this bodily change gives me an idea for another experiment in mindfulness. I ask Kyle if I can say some words to him. He nods. I invite Kyle to get mindful again and to notice what happens when I say, "Your sexual power is welcome here." Kyle reports that something clamps down in his chest. He observes some anger as he stays with the clamping and eventually realizes that underneath the anger, are feelings of grief.

Kyle tells me he wishes he had a different man than his father to model himself after, someone kind and also sexually empowered. I ask if he knows anyone like that. His colleague, Jim, comes to mind. Before we close, I encourage Kyle to go back in time and imagine spending time with a man like Jim when Kyle was a boy. Kyle reports that his belly releases and his spine gets straighter. It feels very different from sucking in his energy. We take time for Kyle to "photograph" this new way of experiencing himself.

During our next session, Kyle acknowledges that Sienna was the first woman he felt he could bring his full sexuality to when he made love. She was sexually expressive and evidently satisfied with the sex they were having. However, when Sienna went into menopause two years ago, her sexuality changed considerably. Penetration was painful, and she needed more active stimulation from Kyle to become fully aroused.

Kyle admits this scared him. He had previously enjoyed a relatively hands-off sex life because Sienna openly masturbated when she needed more stimulation. Now, with the added pressure to stimulate his wife, Kyle wonders if he even knows how. Moreover, whenever Kyle sees what he interprets as Sienna's displeasure, he is overtaken by shame. He feels the familiar impulse to "get sex over with" so as not to burden Sienna, or else he shuts down.

Sienna had no idea that these were Kyle's motives for rushing through sex without pleasuring her. She had only felt blamed for doing something that caused Kyle to lose his arousal. They were missing each other's signals completely. Nor had Kyle realized how much he depended on Sienna to feel confident sexually. Without her enthusiastic expressions, Kyle felt like he was back in college—clueless and insecure.

The psychologist David Schnarch uses the term "borrowed functioning," to describe Kyle's reliance on Sienna to feel like a "good enough" lover.[27] Without Sienna's constant affirmation, Kyle's anxiety would cause him to shut down or withdraw from sex. Kyle suspects that if he didn't feel so much shame around sex, he could ask for feedback instead of dreading each encounter. He might be more willing to check in with Sienna to see what is going on with her when she is making that face.

Sienna reassures Kyle that her displeasure is not with him. The discontent he reads in her pinched face is with her loss of responsiveness. She loves sex and loves having it with him. However, Sienna also feels like she is losing a core part of her identity and is unhappy about that. I ask Kyle to notice that in front of him is a living, breathing woman who has always had a drive equal to or possibly greater than his own. He pauses to take this in.

Sienna continues, "I would love for you to help me discover my changing body. Your teenage self can watch or have a turn, too, and I will let you know what feels especially good to me." Kyle feels self-conscious but also likes the idea. They agree to have a few "discovery sessions" during which Sienna will welcome Kyle's natural sexual curiosity. These sessions enable Kyle to wire in a "missing experience" from his early life. They are also a way to plant hearts, which I will discuss later in the chapter.

## There's an Arrow in Our Tire: Stop-Study-Share

With the examples of Kyle and Sienna and Eric and Max, you can see how I work in session with the befriend cycle, using mindful coinvestigation and mindful self-study. These skills help couples investigate a particular reaction or hidden factor that is inhibiting their sexual life in some way.[28] However, the work doesn't stop here; it requires ongoing attention to the emotional currents within and between both partners when they make love. To this end, I teach couples a simple three-step process to use at home when they get triggered during sex. The technique is called stop-study-share, and is the essence of sexual "response-agility."

Let's go through each step together.

### STEP 1: STOP

Many couples believe they have to go "all the way" if they make or accept sexual advances. However, sex is not an express train: you can stop and get off whenever you want. It is only "by disrupting our habitual behaviors that we open to the possibility of new and creative ways of responding to our wants and fears," writes Tara Brach.[29]

If you are scared of your emotional reactions during sex, you may have developed the habit of pushing ahead when you are uncomfortable. Unfortunately, this will only strengthen your avoidance tendencies around sex. Remember, in the approach of Passion and Presence we use sex not only for pleasure and release but also for healing; "both/and" is the mantra. For this reason, you must agree to pause when either of you is triggered.

Next, it is crucial to get used to stopping so that when you do need to stop, it will be natural to do so. Just as it is hard to be mindful and compassionate at the moment when we are angry, it is hard to pause when we need to. The more we practice mindful awareness, the more such states are available to us in real situations. If we pause whenever we are distracted or losing aliveness during sex, we are building a positive habit to stop when we have an emotional blowout.

The following "drill" builds safety for both partners and can be fun and connecting. It is especially helpful if one of you is afraid of your emotional reactions during sex. Start by setting a timer for forty-five seconds and engage physically in a way that feels good to you both. Agree to pause whenever the timer goes off, whether you need to or not. It is fine to keep this activity under five minutes.

Also, I encourage you to identify a word or signal for stopping whenever you notice you are triggered or that something is dampening your erotic vitality. Here are a few phrases participants in my retreats have come up with:

"I need a moment."

"Something just happened to me, and I'd like to study it."

"Oh wow, I just got activated. Can you do it again so I can notice what happens for me?" (This is mindful coinvestigation.)

"Let's pause. I can sense some sadness is wanting to take me over."

"The 'wait-a-minute' vine just hooked me. I need to back up to unhook."

Identify a word, such as "lemon," or "ouch."

Tap your fingers or make an agreed-upon sound.

## STEP 2: STUDY

As mentioned above, our emotional reactions are fast and automatic. When we are triggered, we may be aware, without knowing why, that we are irritated, whereas moments earlier, we were aroused. We might assume the problem lies with our partner—they aren't doing the right thing to stimulate us. Instead of understanding our reaction, our theories can take us away from our present experience and trap us in the defend cycle.

As we have seen with Eric and Kyle, we can instead find out what our body "knows" by staying with our clenched neck or jaw. If we linger with our body sensations in an open, curious way, we stimulate the neural circuits associated with our emotional memory.[30] Through mindful self-study, we might discover that a rule to avoid showing an interest in sex is hovering just outside of awareness. And that it is the rule, rather than our partner, that is shutting down our sexual excitement.

## STEP 3: SHARE

I encourage you to make a habit of reporting on your discoveries just as we did in the last chapter. Sharing is how we become intimate and undefended. What's more, shame thrives in its own company and dissolves when it's witnessed compassionately by another human being.[31] Being heard by a kind, non-blaming other can be enormously healing.

Sharing is not risk-free, however, and can lead to a breakdown if either of you feels blamed. These exchanges are delicate, which is why it is essential to talk about yourself rather than about your partner. You want to share discoveries about your inner emotional life, even if your reaction was triggered by something your partner said or did. When we can share our experience without blaming our partner, in turn, our partner is likely to provide a caring response.

After completing these three steps, you and your partner can decide whether to:

1. Resume having sex;
2. Adjust before returning, based on your discovery; or
3. Stop and do something else.

Your adjustment may involve making eye contact, shifting your position, hearing reassuring words, changing the temperature in the room, putting on different music, slowing down, moving a hand to another body part, breathing together, or anything that will help you feel present, safe, and connected. Eventually, you may be able to go through the stop-study-share sequence in seconds. For now, agree to give yourselves plenty of time to practice all three steps.

## Turning the Lights On: Seeing Our Habits and Tendencies Clearly

Though the black light syndrome unmasks our hidden factors unexpectedly and often abruptly, our PEP-limiting imprints can also reveal themselves in more subtle ways, such as when we hold ourselves back from expressing our impulses and desires. We can start to practice mindful sex by observing our habits with regard to initiating sex, receiving pleasure, expressing pleasure, and giving pleasure. Because of our ingrained habitual reactions, we may find that we are more comfortable with some of these aspects of sex than others. It is by paying attention that we bring these usually hidden factors into the light.

Jerome and Keisha came to therapy to work on their sexual connection and ended up working on hidden factors as well. During one of our sessions, Keisha complains that Jerome used to be a fun and experimental partner but now lies on his back while she does all the work. Jerome agrees there is some truth to this but has no idea why he is so passive. In his fantasies, he actively pleasures Keisha and has sex in multiple positions.

Jerome agrees to try an experiment in mindfulness. He and Keisha lie on their backs on a floor cushion in my office. Jerome notices that his arms already feel somewhat frozen and that his entire body is becoming tense. I invite Jerome to bring to mind something soothing and comforting. He thinks of his dog, Prince, who is a loyal friend and protector.

When Jerome's breathing relaxes again, I instruct him to get mindful and then to roll onto his side to face Keisha very slowly. I tell him to pay careful attention to anything that changes inside of him as he does so. When Jerome starts turning toward Keisha, he reports that he feels very "strange" and a bit nauseous. He also has the urge to turn away. Since Jerome is able to stay curious, we continue with the experiment. If he was overwhelmed by this feeling, I would stop the experiment at once.

We repeat the sequence a few times, while Jerome studies the "strange" sensation. The third time we do this, Jerome sees an image of his younger brother, Willy. As children, he and Willy shared a bed in their small home in South Carolina. Jerome remembers lying next to Willy, trying to keep himself very still. He suddenly realizes this is the same feeling he has when he is having sex with Keisha.

Jerome puts a hand on his forehead and appears to be troubled. He shakes his head and sighs. "You're remembering something?" I ask, but my question is more of a statement. "And, it's tough to talk about." He nods, and says he's never told anyone about it. I ask what he imagines will happen if he tells us. He pauses and then says, "You'll think I'm a horrible person." "Oh, then I can see why you wouldn't want to tell," I say gently, adding, "I also see that you are in pain." Jerome starts to cry.

Keisha reaches for him and says, "Baby, I love you, that won't change." Jerome takes a breath and then shares the following memory: When Jerome was twelve years old, he woke up in the middle of the night with ejaculate on his fingers and pajamas. He was on his knees facing Willy. Jerome had no idea what happened, and still doesn't, but he was flooded with dread and shame. He felt that it was his job to keep Willy safe and that he failed him miserably.

When I ask Jerome what his younger self is learning from this experience, he pauses to feel into this and then says, "I can't trust myself," and "I have to be very careful, or I will hurt the people I love." "Oh," I say softly, sounding mildly surprised. "And, given that you carry this 'truth' inside, what do you do?" Jerome tells me that from then on, he always kept himself very still when he was lying beside Willy, especially when he was older and felt aroused. He learned how to sleep in the same position and not to move at all at night.

Jerome had no idea that a part of himself was still afraid of violating the person in his bed because the hidden factors operate automatically, outside of awareness. He now sees that he has been relying on the same strategy of "staying passive" with Keisha. I turn to Keisha who is visibly moved by this story. She reaches for Jerome and holds him as tears run down both of their cheeks. She tells him how sorry she feels that young Jerome suffered from this secret and that she now understands why he holds himself back during sex.

## To Thine Own Heart Be True

Scientists have discovered that when old memories like this one are activated, they are plastic for a four-hour window.[32] If healing experiences imprint during this window, we can extinguish the emotional learning connected to a distressing memory, though not the memory itself.

It works like this: When you have an unpleasant feeling or reaction, stay with it long enough for an image or memory to surface that helps you understand its origin. When you have a sense of the original imprint, and the feeling tone of the wound is active, you and your partner can design a way to give you something now that you would have needed back then to move through life with an intact sexual identity.

For example, if you received an unwanted touch one or more times in the past, and it left you with a bad feeling about yourself or sex, you can pair the "live" memory of that experience with a touch that feels considerate, respectful, and pleasing *right now*. I call this activity "planting a heart." It involves encoding a corrective experience provided by your partner to transform a sexual wound from the past.

All of us have PEP-limiting imprints planted in the seedbed of our erotic life. When we plant a new seed beside an old one (i.e., a "heart"), they graft together, and the resulting tree bears sweeter fruit. The scientific term for this process is *memory reconsolidation*.[33] When we receive a heart, we erase the emotional learning connected to our suffering. Instead of operating from limiting, unconscious patterns, options emerge that didn't exist before.

As another example, if the experience of unwanted touch generated a belief that you have to endure things that don't feel good to you, then you can design an activity in which you get to say, "stop" or "remove your hand," and your partner does so. In this instance, the heart is something of a do-over of the first experience with an empowering outcome.

I have done the heart-planting exercise with countless couples in my retreats and private practice. Couples are always amazed that planting hearts works so well and that they know just what they need to experience from their partner to repair past wounds. Here are some examples of different kinds of hearts:

Putting their partner's hand on their genitals in a safe and
connecting way to affirm that having sexual feelings is okay
A do-over of something that went wrong, such as "playing
doctor"
Receiving protection, in the form of being hidden from
unwanted attention
Being able to remove an unwanted touch or say no, as in the
example above
Having the ability to give consent (or not) before being
touched to repair an earlier boundary intrusion
Going slow and checking in continuously to counter the
experience of being overpowered in the past
Hearing words like, "I love your breasts" (or any part of the
body that brings shame), or "It's natural to be curious

about your genitals" (for example, speaking to a younger part of oneself that was caught masturbating)

After Jerome unburdens his secret, Jerome and Keisha agree to plant hearts. I encourage Jerome to let the feeling that he is unsafe for others to retake hold. Accessing the emotional "takeaway" of the original experience prepares the soil so the heart will take root. Keisha then tells Jerome that she feels completely safe with him, especially sexually. He looks into her eyes and can sense this is true. I invite him to notice what happens in his body as he senses the truth of this. He describes warmth in his chest and tingling in his arms, which feel pleasurable. He realizes that his arms had previously felt frozen. I encourage Jerome to stay with the pleasant sensations and make a "photograph" of the aliveness in his arms.

During sex, Jerome and Keisha begin actively teaming to transform old wounds by planting hearts. Jerome pauses whenever he notices he is tensing or becoming passive. At those times, Keisha reminds him that he is a grown man now, and this is what consenting adults do. Also, whenever Jerome makes sounds, reaches for Keisha, or moves in new ways, Keisha tells him that she feels completely safe and enjoys receiving his full sexual aliveness. Jerome is becoming increasingly open and expressive, as he and Keisha plant hearts to transform the belief that "I have to be careful," to "It's safe to be sexually free."

Figure 4.4, "The 5 Ss," shows all five steps for working with and transforming the hidden factors as a couple. Steps 1, 2, and 3 are stop, study, share. Step 4 is "select." Here is where you decide whether to stop the encounter, for now, adjust and resume, or plant a heart. Step 5 is to savor the good feelings connected to whichever choice you make and teaming up to heal and grow.

## THINGS THAT GO BUMP IN THE NIGHT: EROTIC WOUNDING AND TRAUMA

One does not become enlightened by imagining figures of light, but by making the darkness conscious.
—C. J. Jung[34]

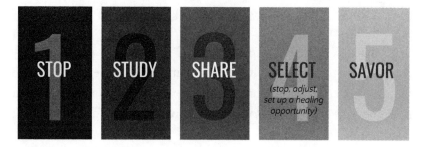

**FIGURE 4.4 THE 5 Ss**

The 5 Ss are a path and practice for working with the hidden factors. We **stop, study,** and **share** whenever we are triggered or losing aliveness. Then we select from the following options: adjust and resume, plant a heart, or agree to end the encounter. Finally, we **savor** the good feelings resulting from whichever option we select.

## The Darkest Imprints

No matter how open our family or sensitive our first lover, somewhere along the line we likely experienced hurt and shame around sexuality, creating erotic wounding, and possibly trauma. These are the darkest form of imprints. Trauma can damage our sexual identity, leading us to feel broken and ashamed. When it comes to sex, we may be afraid of being overwhelmed by the experience or flooded by intrusive memories when we have it.

In my experience, trauma survivors suffer two kinds of abuse. The first is the original wound, while the second and more insidious injury is the disparaging way we may view ourselves as "damaged goods." Many trauma survivors feel like sexual failures when they aren't able to do what our culture considers to be "real" sex.

The concept of pure erotic potential can be especially helpful in these circumstances. If you remember, satisfying sex has little to do with what you do in bed and everything to do with your state of mind. As we have seen, the performance trance tells us we have to match our behavior to what our culture considers to be "functional" sex to be worthy. This idea is nonsense. You can access your pure erotic potential right now merely by turning toward pleasure.

Pleasure may or may not involve genital contact, penetration, or orgasm. When I encourage trauma survivors to discover their own pathways to pleasure by going "off script," their relief is palpable. They come alive with the possibility of connecting through their bodies again in nonthreatening ways. This is why I view non-goal sex as a freedom movement. It is freedom from the tyranny of outside-in definitions of healthy, normal, or hot sex.

Unfortunately, in cases of unresolved trauma, some part of us may be frozen back in time, unaware that we are no longer in the original experience.[35] If this is true for you, you will want to find a trauma therapist to help you heal and become safely embodied again.[36]

## Going Off Script: Six Ways to Detach Now from Then

If you have already begun your healing journey and have professional support, the following six steps may make having sex a safer and more enjoyable experience for you:

1. Let go of goals, models, and reference points
2. Become alert to your body's signals of pleasure and discomfort
3. Say something when you are moving into an unpleasant state
4. Pause to study what is happening
5. Introduce a change so you are not reenacting an earlier experience
6. Design and then savor a transformational experience

Let's go through these steps with Sue, a retreat participant who also met with me for three individual sessions. Sue is a forty-seven-year-old survivor of childhood sexual abuse married to a towering "gentle giant" named Barney. Barely five feet tall, Sue has a sparkling personality and warm smile, and is eager to feel safe and expressive during sex.

In 2012, Sue spent a month at a treatment center for trauma. While Sue believes her treatment was lifesaving, she can still have times when she freezes or is gripped during sex, and she occasionally shuts down when Barney climaxes. Sue and Barney came to our couple's Passion and Presence retreat because Sue felt that mindfulness would help her develop a more trusting relationship with her body—and it did.

## 1. LET GO OF GOALS, MODELS, AND REFERENCE POINTS

Sue was able to recognize that she was preoccupied with the idea that she had to become aroused to ready herself for intercourse. This performance mind-set was interfering with her ability to relax and let go. I reminded Sue of the danger of models, especially when they become a reference point while we make love. She agreed to relinquish her goal-directed agenda and to open to the experience unfolding between her and Barney.

## 2. BECOME ALERT TO YOUR BODY'S SIGNALS OF PLEASURE AND DISCOMFORT

Sue spent years feeling guilty and ashamed because, as a child, she felt pleasure within the complex mix of emotions related to her abuse. I explained that our bodies are designed to respond to sexual stimulation, automatically—whether we consent to it or not. Research indicates that, for women, lubricating when exposed to sexual stimuli has an evolutionary advantage: it protects them from injury and infection during unwanted penetration.[37]

Nevertheless, Sue felt betrayed by her body for doing what nature intended it to do. As an adult, she managed feelings of shame by distracting herself to avoid feeling anything during sex. Reversing this habit took time, patience, and self-compassion. Mindfulness and body scan exercises are now a vital part of Sue's efforts to become safely embodied.

Both of these practices help cultivate "somatic self-attunement," which allows us to use information from our bodies to guide us toward pleasure and away from anything that feels harmful or toxic. When we form this kind of attuned relationship with ourselves, protection can grow through wakefulness rather than guardedness. We can honor our limits by decoding our body's signals for yes and no rather than by establishing blanket rules such as "never touch me here," or "don't make that sound."

Rules make sense when other people are violating our boundaries. Here, in this time and place, Sue had created a safe relationship with a loving and caring partner, so she no longer needed the same set of rules. She now has many more resources than she did as a child. Thus, what was dangerous, disempowering, and shameful back then might be experienced differently at this stage of life. Sue liked hearing this.

Just as eroticism is always changing, so are we. Through cultivating somatic self-attunement, we can adjust our parameters accordingly. When we feel our bandwidth is broad, we might decide to go toward our erotic edge. If we feel our bandwidth is narrow, we may need to limit the length and type of contact we have for today. When our relationship is grounded in response-agility, as Sue's and Barney's was, we can pause and adjust to fit our changing capacities from one moment to the next.

### 3. SAY SOMETHING WHEN YOU ARE MOVING INTO AN UNPLEASANT STATE

Sadly, Sue, like many abuse survivors, had to keep her experience a secret. Many survivors were blamed when they sought help, or they had no one to talk to about their abuse. Until recently, Sue was repeating this silencing by trying to manage moments of fear and pain alone. Barney could feel that Sue seemed distracted, but he interpreted her lack of presence as being due to work-related stress. Now, Sue is pausing to partner with Barney; they are making adjustments as needed to be safely connected.

### 4. PAUSE TO STUDY WHAT IS HAPPENING

Sue was comfortable when Barney was tender, but when his arousal led to the plateau stage, before orgasm, his involuntary movements scared her. The couple decided to design an experiment using mindful coinvestigation in which Barney made involuntary movements in a goofy, nonsexual context. Before the investigation began, however, Sue noticed that she was already feeling tense.

As she stayed with the sensation of gripping her muscles, she noticed energy coursing through her right arm. She continued to study her body sensations and found she wanted to push Barney away. This natural "fight" reaction was compromised during the abuse, but Sue's body was still longing to express this essential survival strategy.[38]

Sue and Barney paused to explore how they might plant a heart. What could they do in this moment to install a reparative experience? Sue went into a mindful state and realized she wanted the experience of pushing her abuser, Justin, away. To enjoy her sexuality, she needed to recover a sense of personal power that was missing for most of her life.

Going slow, and feeling the muscles involved with pushing, Sue let herself push Barney. At first, Barney resisted a bit too much, but at Sue's request, he allowed his arms to be pushed away. They repeated the successful pushing activity a few times until Sue fell onto her knees, exhausted but satisfied with herself.[39]

Sue and Barney decided to go a step further and "uncouple" Justin from Barney. They spent a few minutes looking into each other's eyes, and Sue was able to recognize that Barney was a kind and gentle man who had never misused his power with her. Barney held Sue for a long time so Sue could feel a sense of safety in his arms. Several times, she asked Barney to release his arms so she could experience a sense of control. After a while, Sue could feel her body un-grip. With a deep sigh, she surrendered into herself, and into Barney's arms.

A note of caution needs to be offered here. Mindful coinvestigation can bring up strong feelings because you are introducing a triggering stimulus. Sue had already done these exercises under close supervision. If you find that you are experiencing "too much, too fast," back off from the activity. Find a way to stay safely connected, perhaps lying on your sides facing one another.

## 5. INTRODUCE A CHANGE SO YOU ARE NOT REENACTING AN EARLIER EXPERIENCE

Sue realized that gripping was her automatic strategy to deal with feeling overpowered. She decided to take her gripping as a cue to make a small adjustment. Often this meant finding a way to have more space between her and Barney. Sometimes she needed to ask him to release his arms or shift positions. All of these things he was glad to do, which continued to help Sue detach now from then.

If we are present, we can listen to ourselves every step of the way. Mindfulness can help us notice when something feels off course. At such times, we can discern whether we need to stop or merely adjust what we are doing. Stopping, studying, and adjusting is how we recover the control that was missing in the past.

## 6. DESIGN AND THEN SAVOR
## A TRANSFORMATIONAL EXPERIENCE

Like Sue's "numbing" and "gripping," we develop protective strategies to manage our experience. These are creative and necessary safeguards against reinjury. Unfortunately, we may use these strategies whether we need them or not. For instance, if you learned to dissociate when you were younger, then you are likely to always dissociate, out of habit, whether anything dangerous is happening or not. As a result, in all probability you don't notice opportunities for safety, mutuality, connection, and pleasure that may be available today because you aren't here for them.

Sue felt helpless and disempowered during the abuse, and her internal model was, "People will dominate me," "It is fruitless to resist," and "I cause others to lose control." As a five-year-old child, those beliefs were not conscious thoughts; they were a "truth" encoded in her felt sense. Unbeknownst to Sue, these truths, or hidden factors, were still guiding her behavior.

The good news is that we can bring ourselves up to date. We are in a different world now, filled with possible reparative experiences. However, if our focus is pointed elsewhere, we will undoubtedly miss them. As we have seen, neuroscience tells us that by training our attention we can rewire our brain. When we notice and integrate reparative experiences, we harness the brain's neuroplasticity.[40]

For example, if our partner stops when we ask them to stop, and we pay attention to the new and different experience, we can rewire the belief, "I'm not safe," to "I'm safe right now," or, "I'm safe with Barney." If my partner checks in with me during sex, I can rewire the belief that "I'll be exploited if I open up" to, "I'm open, and I'm being cared for." For this internal rewiring to happen, we must be present to savor the emotional and somatic *experience* of the new belief.[41]

Barney wanted to participate in Sue's recovery and do everything in his power to help Sue detach now from then. For this reason, he suggested they set up an experiment wherein Sue could experience a sense of control and safety in a sexual context. Sue loved this idea but wasn't sure how to create such an experience or whether it would work. However, just feeling Barney's support gave her a deeply healing sense of being a team. The burden shifted from Sue having to heal herself, alone, to teaming up to create experiences to restore her sense of safety and her enjoyment of sex.

After some discussion, they decided to engage physically and for Sue to stop whenever she needed to adjust, and also to savor experiences of pleasure and connection. In addition, Barney agreed to tell Sue what he wanted to do before doing it and to ask for consent. While committed couples often skip the formality of asking for permission, time and again, I have found that doing so creates safety for both people with and without a trauma history.

Sue and Barney shared the story of their experience with me. They begin with five minutes of mindfulness practice focusing on their breathing bodies. They notice where the breath seems to originate from and let their attention rest in that area. As they sense the rise and fall of each breath, they pay attention to the expansion and release in different parts of their bodies. They are not trying to manufacture a good state—they simply let awareness move throughout the body as it breathes. When they drift into thinking or anticipation, they gently return to the breath, letting thoughts and fantasies go so they can be right here, in this moment.

In the next phase of the exercise, they look into each other's eyes. Sue takes a moment to see Barney and says to herself what she agreed before the exercise would be most helpful. "This is Barney, not Justin." Sue lets herself be present to the truth in front of her. Barney asks if he can stroke her face. Sue consents and is feeling the sensation of Barney's hand on her skin, as he wipes back some hair that has fallen onto her face. Barney asks if it is okay to move a finger across her eyelid and Sue nods. Then he cups the back of her neck as if to draw her in for a kiss. Sue is feeling all of this and notices that the cupping creates a bit of the trapped feeling she typically endures. Instead, she decides to make an adjustment. She asks Barney to remove his hand. Sue lets herself appreciate that Barney honors her request.

Sue says to herself, "He is stopping when I say no! He is checking in with me and not just focusing on himself." Sue tells Barney that she wants to pause to feel the truth of this in her body. She shares, "My breath deepens, and my pelvis unlocks. Let me savor this good feeling." Pausing and experiencing is how we help a heart to grow roots.

After forty seconds or so, Sue opens her eyes and looks at Barney again. He is looking back at her. He tells her how much he loves her. Internally, Sue says, "Barney is looking at me and using my name. He is seeing me right now as a real person and not an object. Let me pause to notice what it is like to be in contact during sex." She asks if they can just breathe together. Barney agrees. It is crucial to create a sense of safety by going slowly. Otherwise, old strategies of protection will switch on automatically.

Barney asks Sue if he can kiss the backs of her hands. She consents. Barney has learned a few phrases to help Sue stay with her felt experience. He asks her to notice what happens in her body. Sue reports "I notice I come into my body more. I feel warmth on my skin where you placed your hand. Let me bathe in that." Then, Barney strokes her right arm. Sue takes his hand and puts it on her shoulder instead. He smiles and nods.

Internally, Sue says, "Wow, my preferences matter to Barney. He isn't upset at all that I asked him to remove his hand from my arm. We are a team. We are adjusting to fit my needs. Wait. Let me really get this." "This is different," Sue says aloud, "I like feeling that we are a team. I feel more grown up. Oh, my neck just got longer, and my hips feel more solid. Let me take a moment to feel how it is to feel my grown-up body with you." Sue compares the grown-up feeling of teaming to the child-like experience of being alone and overpowered. This truly is different. Sue smiles. Barney smiles back. He repeats, "I love you and you are safe now." He encourages her to notice that.

Sue is suddenly very touched. Her eyes water. Internally, the words come into her head that "Barney actually values my sexuality, and I feel respected and cared for. Let me breathe that in too. We are kind to each other. I can go slow. As I know that, I can feel more turn on in my body. I feel safe right now. I am in my capacity. I can enjoy the pleasure I feel in my genitals and down through my toes. Oh, that's fun—my toes are pulsing a bit."

Barney asks, "What else is different right now?" Sue pauses and says, "There is no manipulation here, you are asking permission. I can stop anytime." He nods and encourages Sue to savor this difference. Sue tells Barney that she's had enough for now. They hold each other skin to skin. Sue tells herself, "I feel Barney's erection, but he doesn't need anything from me. He's just here with me. I am safe."

Sue and Barney had several of these "detaching" sessions for a few weeks. Sue used these sessions to "lock in" experiences of safety, control, and trust. She learned that Barney can control himself around her and that she can let go instead of needing to stay gripped when they are erotic together. As a result, Sue is starting to enjoy sex in ways that weren't possible before.

As a team activity, it is important that these experiments be co-constructed and that you and your partner establish clear guidelines for the intent, length, and process you will use during a detaching session. Please remember it is important to go slow, and to ensure there is adequate time for pausing to savor the corrective experience.

## It's Tea for Two: Trauma Is a Couple's Issue

So far, we've been focusing on the survivor. However, if you are the partner of a survivor, you may feel:

Rejected and sexually deprived
Guilty for wanting sex
Grief and resentment because you cannot have a
    "normal" sex life
Judged and ashamed for wanting sex
Guilty or blamed when your partner gets triggered
Helpless at supporting your partner
Cautious about triggering your partner

Reluctant to initiate

Fearful of being "too much"

Tense and contained during sex

While Barney was sad that Sue struggled and was mad at her abuser, he did not suffer when Sue declined his invitations for sex. However, Sam, another retreat participant who identifies as non-binary, felt that inhibiting their desires restimulated their old wounds. As a child, Sam was hindered by their overbearing mother whenever they wanted anything. They felt repeatedly denied of things that were important to them and restricted by their mother's expectations—especially when it came to their gender identity. That experience was painful to their younger self and left them feeling disempowered even today. Not surprisingly, Sam feels resentful when their partner, Wren, a trauma survivor, repeatedly rejects their sexual advances.

A team approach to healing through sex recognizes that the hidden factors are shaping the experiences of *both* partners. The feelings of rejection triggered in Sam when Wren says no, coupled with feeling thwarted, are a product of Sam's imprint portfolio. Sam's wounds automatically open when Wren pushes them away.

Sam explains that they struggled for a long time to feel a sense of belonging. It was years before they knew the term "gender dysphoria," and even longer before they recognized its contribution to their struggles with depression. They didn't feel accepted at home, and their mother's repeated attempts to mold them into someone they didn't want to be left them feeling empty and unwanted. Sam wondered if they would ever have a satisfying sexual relationship before meeting Wren, a cisgender woman who was completely accepting of Sam's non-binary gender identity.

Wren tells me that she has had other genderqueer partners and has explored different avenues of her own sexuality. She is an advocate for shedding the idea that one person assumes the active role while the other is passive and receptive during sex. This dominance and submission template is an example of gender essentialism,[42] Wren says. She seems passionate about the subject.

Unfortunately, Wren's progressive views on sexuality have not erased the imprint of her early abuse or other hidden factors from her past. It is for this reason that black light syndrome can be so beguiling. Consciously, we may have sex-positive attitudes and actively promote them; however, in the bedroom, our expressed ideas about sex and our tacit somatic knowing don't always line up. Wren admits that despite her efforts to support sexual empowerment, she still has an aversive reaction to being touched in certain places and gets easily triggered by sex. At the same time, it pains Wren to hurt Sam by saying no to sex more often than yes. Moreover, Wren insists that she is eager to heal from her abuse and detach *now* from *then*.

Both want to do right by the other. After exploring this impasse, and its impact on Sam in particular, they came up with a creative way to honor Wren's need for safety and Sam's longing for a sense of sexual agency. Sam and Wren agreed to schedule dates in which Wren will use somatic self-attunement to identify a part of her body that Sam can freely explore without fear of reprisal from Wren. They designed this activity in a spirit of cooperation, rather than a businesslike quid pro quo.

A few months later, they reported that the experiment was working: Wren is setting boundaries using her growing capacity to sense what her body needs at the moment. With mindfulness, she is learning to differentiate between the discomfort of doing something new and the danger of doing something harmful. Consequently, she is more confident in expanding her limits when it feels safe to do so.

For Sam, hearing "yes" rather than "no" is affirming on multiple fronts. It is giving Sam a sense of acceptance more directly and powerfully than through words alone, along with the intimate contact that was missing from their profoundly loving relationship.

By teaming up to plant hearts, Sam and Wren moved through a painful impasse that was also preventing them from growing. Both are transforming old imprints by using what had been coming between them to heal and grow.

## MINDFUL ACTIVITIES AND NAKED REFLECTIONS

. . . . . . . . . . . . . . . . . . . . . . . . . . . . . . . . . . . . . . . . . . . . . . . . . . . . . .

## Mindful Self-Study (10–20 minutes)

. . . . . . . . . . . . . . . . . . . . . . . . . . . . . . . . . . . . . . . . . . . . . . . . . . . . . .

Each person in the partnership should complete this exercise separately at a time when you are not rushed and are unlikely to be interrupted.

*Step 1: Take 2 minutes to enter a mindful state.*

*Step 2: Let yourself touch into an unpleasant emotion related to sex.*

*Step 3: Try to activate it by lingering with the emotion with curiosity.*

What starts to happen as you touch into this? Allow all feelings, body sensations, and images to show up that go with this emotion. Give yourself at least a couple of minutes for this lingering.

*Step 4: After several minutes of feeling into yourself, you may have memories of events or people you were involved with. Reflect on what this reaction seems to thread to in your history.*

It may not even be a sexual thing, but rather some knowledge you carry about what is and isn't okay. Look for examples.

If no memory appears, study what your body/mind seems to have learned.

*Step 5: Sense the imprints you carry and how this "knowing" has played out in your life, with your partner, or in past relationships.*

Don't push to connect the dots. Be open to what is unfolding in your experience as you linger with curiosity and acceptance.

Sharing: When you are complete, share your discoveries with your partner.

## Planting a Heart (around 15 minutes)

Try this exercise together as a couple. Make sure you both have time and are feeling connected and open to one another. Find a private space and make sure you won't be interrupted. Take time afterward to be together in a kind and loving way.

Planting a heart involves setting up a "do-over" of a painful past event, mainly when the feelings connected to the experience are alive. It is a powerful exercise to do after the stop-study-share activity when an erotic encounter triggers a memory of an actual wound. If the mindful self-study activity generated a painful memory, you could plant a heart around that.

### Step 1: Partner A

While staying present to the activation, (which may mean with your eyes closed as in mindful self-study), ask yourself, or have your partner ask you these questions:

#### The Wound

What feelings do I carry from this experience?
What did I learn about myself, others, and sexuality?
What kind of limiting belief did I imprint from this experience?

#### Identifying the Heart

What would have helped me feel okay back then (or safe, desirable, worthy, normal)?
What would have empowered me to claim my sexuality as a beautiful part of myself?
What did I need from another at the time?
What kind of heart do I want now? (Some possibilities are kindness, interest, comfort, touch, words, protection, and help understanding why that happened.)

### Step 2: Both Partners

Codesign a way to offer this experience (i.e., the "heart") right now.

### Step 3: Partner A

Get mindful in preparation for the heart. This mindful interlude is an important step to ensure the heart takes root.

### Step 4: Partner A

Call up the part of you that was wounded and put yourself in that experience again. Remember how it felt and the painful emotional takeaway. When ready to receive the heart, nod your head.

### Step 5: Partner B

Offer the heart to partner A.

### Savor the Heart

If the heart feels good, imagine anchoring your new heart in the soil by taking at least two minutes to enjoy the good feelings you are experiencing. Receive the heart again, if desired.

If the heart is not quite right, make adjustments as needed until it is "good enough" for Partner A. Repeat steps 3 and 4 before offering the heart again.

### Step 6: Both Partners

Connect lovingly and find a way to complete the activity. Switch roles if desired.

## Naked Reflections

Explore how you feel about yourself and your partner, having completed this activity. How has this wound shown up in your sex life as a couple? Are you willing to cultivate response-agility as a team (i.e., shifting from making love to researching triggers as needed?) How can planting hearts support your healing and deepening as an erotic team?

# 5.

## EROTIC EXPRESSION

### Overcoming Shame to Reclaim
### Your Full Self

When you suppress any part of your eroticism, you
suppress nothing short of your full aliveness.
—JOY DAVIDSON[1]

In the action comedy *Date Night*, a "boring couple from New Jersey"
(the Fosters) take on a new identity and fall madly, passionately in love
all over again.[2] How does this happen? Each discovers that their beloved
is much more complex and multidimensional than the person they go
on date night with week after week.

In the opening act, we see parts of them that we might name the
"exhausted nine-to-fiver," "prudish spectator," "repressed lover," "nice
guy," and "responsible spouse." These parts interact in predictably
hypnotic ways. However, when the couple assumes a new identity
(the Tripplehorns), the singularly upright pair discover their inner
"superhero" and also their "tough guy," "pimp," "stripper," "flirt," and
"burglar" parts.

Erotic expression happens in two dimensions: there is *what* we
do, or the kind of sexual experience we are seeking, and *who* we are
when we have sex. Let's start with the "who." Like the Fosters, all of
us have a variety of parts or subpersonalities that appear inside and

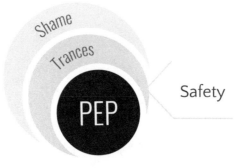

FIGURE 5.1 CHAPTER 5 PEP BARRIERS

outside of the bedroom. Some are "nice" while others are "naughty." "I will always be the virgin-prostitute, the perverse angel, the two-faced sinister and saintly woman," writes Anaïs Nin.[3] Accordingly, a mindful approach is accepting of all of these characters. It is "both/and," and not sanctimonious.

While we may have brought these parts into the bedroom at stage 1, by the time we hit stage 2 many of us feel so typecast in our role of mother/father, wife/husband/partner, or worker that we can't access anyone else during sex. We end up putting eros in a box that is much too small for this dynamic, life-giving force. Why do we make such a tradeoff? Is it fear of rejection—of exposing our hidden shame—that leads us to fall into a sexual script that we can safely follow? Or do we become increasingly risk-averse in our trade of thrilling nights for a secure future together?

Indeed, many stage 2 couples report an internal conflict between fulfilling their adult responsibilities and being free, even wild. Instead of expressing our "sovereign power," as Davidson calls it,[4] we may tamp down our aliveness so that, in bed, the image of a respectable grown-up—as a spouse, parent, and wage earner—hijacks eros. Alternatively, we may flit between being "good" and being secretly "naughty" without having a way to integrate both parts of ourselves consciously and expansively.

Carla admits that when her passionate, multifaceted self shrunk to fit her familial obligations, she subsequently lost interest in sex. You may recall from chapter 2, that Carla felt a fire long extinguished in her marriage light up with her coworker, Porsha. For the first time in years, Carla felt life-size, beautiful, and best of all—daring.

A tired relationship with your spouse is hard to compare with the novelty-induced dopamine explosion that comes with a new alliance. Alas, as we have seen, that sense of euphoria will undoubtedly be short-lived. Moreover, breaking out of your sexual straitjacket by having an affair may be one way to feel free, but it also carries a cost. The naked path offers us a genuinely growth-inducing alternative.

Eros carries a powerful urge to express itself in creative and daring ways. We dampen our sex lives by doing the same things over and over, and also by bringing the same *selves* to every encounter.[5] Thus, the trick for staying engaged in a committed relationship is to liberate ourselves from the shrink-to-fit imperative that can cut off our erotic blood supply at stage 2.

Regrettably, like Carla, many of us would sooner find a new lover than *be* a new lover with our long-term partner because of the risks this nakedness entails. Many stage 2 couples I have worked with have fallen into imagining that certain parts of them are unwelcome in the bedroom. We may even fear those parts might trigger our mate in some way. From here, it is easy to slip into a safety trance, where we privilege security over creative expression (see figure 5.2, "Safety Trance"). No wonder some of us feel free only with other partners.

The safety trance convinces us that if we are too wild, or pleasure seeking, that we will imperil our relationship and find ourselves skating on dangerously thin ice. As a result, we follow the straight-and-narrow path of our risk-free yet insufferably dulling routine. Stage 3 couples take the naked path instead. They avoid hiding, shrinking—and sneaking—by taking risks with *each other* and by engaging in what I call whole-person multimodal sex. However, before we dare ourselves to be brave, let's see how shame and the safety trance may be hijacking your aliveness.

## SHAME AS THE LIE

Shame is the lie someone told you about yourself.
—Anaïs Nin[6]

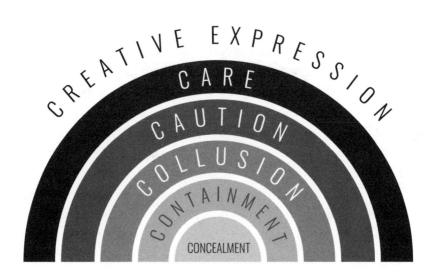

**FIGURE 5.2 SAFETY TRANCE**

In the safety trance, we sacrifice creative expression for security. We avoid any "risky moves" that might rupture our bond. On the path from care to concealment, we hide or numb our erotic impulses, or we engage in covert behaviors to satisfy our unmet needs for expression.

Shame exists in all cultures as part of the socialization process. We learn the codes of conduct in our family and are brought up short when we defy them.[7] Sometimes, this psychic (or physical) whack is for our safety, like when our parents yank our hand away from a sharp object. However, experiences in childhood of being "corrected" can leave a stain if we are not brought back into loving connection soon after.

Brené Brown defines shame as "the intensely painful feeling or experience of believing that we are flawed and therefore unworthy of love and belonging."[8] It can take root for a variety of reasons. For example, as children, being bullied, marginalized, or sexually abused can be damaging, even damning, to our sense of belonging.[9] As adults, a passing smirk or eye roll from our partner can also evoke the steely pain of our shame-filled imprints, as we saw with Eric and Max.

While guilt is a feeling of having done something wretched, shame convinces us that we *are* wretched.[10] When we ingest this lie, we tell ourselves we are ugly, stupid, rotten, bad, disgusting, inadequate, and wrong. As a consequence, feelings of shame warn us to keep our deepest, darkest, most "depraved" thoughts to ourselves, which is how it becomes a self-perpetuating supply chain. Shame reproduces and recharges itself through isolation and secrecy.

The costs of shame are enormous. Like high blood pressure, shame is a silent killer—of eros, dignity, and self-worth. It inhibits us from fully expressing ourselves and can lead us to imagine scenarios of humiliation and failure when we consider taking a risk. Many of us learn to skirt anything that might imperil our sense of belonging.

This strategy explains why we often become increasingly risk-averse both emotionally and sexually after the "magic dust" of our green and passionate relationship begins to settle. Our newly minted relationship is like winning a lottery ticket or feeling like we have found an insurance policy against life as an outcast that has eluded us until now. Why would we do something that might put our security in peril?

Up to now I have been talking about the general feelings of shame that most often have their genesis in early childhood experiences. What makes our intimate relationship so complex is that many of us carry sexual shame on top of a general sense of shame. Thus, we may believe that our desires, fantasies, bodies, genitals, and past deeds are anywhere from embarrassing to appalling. Some of us even experience "a visceral feeling of humiliation and disgust toward our body and identity as a sexual being and a belief of being abnormal and inferior," as Noel Clark describes it.[11]

This belief is hardly surprising given the deep roots of sex-negativity in our society. Nonetheless, you may be astounded to learn that the clinical name for female genitalia, *pudendum*, derives from the verb *pudēre*, which means "to be ashamed."[12] Consider this too: in 1995, President Clinton fired his surgeon general, Jocelyn Elders, for suggesting that teaching masturbation might be an effective way to prevent the spread of AIDS.[13] Until 2003, sixteen states had laws criminalizing oral and anal sex between consenting adults. Today, you can bring your gun to college, but leave your dildo at home unless you want to face jail time in Louisiana, Alabama, or Virginia.[14]

When we come into a relationship with a sense of shame or unworthiness, it is hard to avoid feeling naked at stage 2. Indeed, many of us experience a feeling of worthiness at stage 1 because someone finally sees us as "good"—even *chooses* us. From such a high, it is no wonder the sting of the leaden arrow can provoke such devastation. Hidden feelings of shame and unworthiness can become unleashed, evoking fears that our partner can see through us and see the "bad" person we "really are." We might even believe we could somehow poison our partners if they get too close.

When the golden and intoxicating façade of stage 1 wears off, we can go into legacy states more often and not uncommonly, during sex. Why, then, would we want to expose all of that "badness," even to ourselves, by having sex? When shame shows up in our long-term sexual relationship, as it must, we sometimes flee for the hills and abandon our partner. More often though, we hide in a safe place *within* sex; we limit not just what we can do in bed, but also who we *are* in bed to protect our oasis of security.

We all need belonging: it is our birthright. However, when we obtain this right by hiding who we are, we have no permanent home—in the world, our relationship, or ourselves. For this reason, I invite my clients to start by looking at how shame may have set up patterns of containment when it comes to sex. To support this, it is important to learn to bring nonjudgmental awareness to the fact that for many of us, our safe place may have become our prison.

## SHAME BUSTING AS A LIBERATION MOVEMENT

Honoring diverse sexual appetites and expressions is a necessary antidote to feeling shame about sex. I like to talk about how this honoring is like learning to exercise a "shame-busting muscle." While we often categorize sex as chocolate or vanilla, heteronormative or queer, as the feminist psychoanalyst Suzanne Iasenza points out, all sex is queer.[15] When we resist the urge to create an "us" and a "them,"[16] or a "right" or "wrong," we create a patch of grass for our kind of "different." We make room for the silent, unspoken sexual desires we have no matter how conventional or "outlandish" they may be.

Sexual preferences come in all sizes, shapes, and colors; however, not all identities are created equal. Being socially marginalized (remember the importance of belonging) and a community subjected to hate crimes regularly may explain why 40–50 percent of transgender and gender nonconforming people attempt suicide in their lifetime.[17]

For these reasons and the fact that most of us feel shame around our sexual desires, I have come to view shame busting as a liberation movement that starts at home. While there's still much to do on the geopolitical stage, our private sexual theater can become a shame-free zone, a place where all of our parts can have safe expression.

A starting place is to take conscious measures to triumph over shame rather than to succumb to its pull or—often more damaging— to conspire to avoid it. That is, when we feel shame, our impulse is to contract and pull away, even from ourselves. We may experience physical sensations that accompany these impulses, such as tension in our belly, nausea, tightness in our chest. We might become irritable and withdrawn, or want to attack our partner in some way (remember the "defend cycle").

As we saw in chapter 4, we can set an intention to plant hearts at such moments by meeting ourselves and our partner with compassion. We can go even further and dare ourselves to express rather than hide our desires. Joy Davidson tells us that to absolve ourselves of shame, we can "expose it to the light" or we can "eroticize it."[18] Stage 3 couples create a relational container grounded in *caring* and do both. Firstly, through *sharing*, they openly express their desires ("expose it to the light"). Secondly, by *daring* to integrate parts they have cast to the shadows, they "eroticize" that which they consider shameful.

## THE SAFETY TRANCE: WHEN CARE AND CAUTION BECOME COLLUSION

Undefended intimacy . . . unfolds when we have developed the ability to express all the parts of our being while in a relationship with another who is doing the same.
—Jett Psaris and Marlena S. Lyons[19]

Lots of things can stop us from bringing our full aliveness to our long-term relationship. Sometimes we hide our desires and default to a safe, albeit deadening, script because we don't want to trigger our partner. As we saw in chapter 4, at stage 2, we now know each other's vulnerabilities and will often take care to protect our partner—and ourselves—from triggering them.

The problem with practicing "safe sex" in this way is that we can lose a sense of free-flowing expression, if not lust for life. When we think we have to hide to preserve our connection, we start to dodge each other's sensitive "hot spots" and suppress impulses that diverge from our script. Once we fall into this safety trance, our care can lead from caution to collusion (refer to figure 5.2). That is, if our partner is equally risk-averse, we make a devil's bargain not to upset the apple cart. We often give up any "risky moves" that might jeopardize our feelings of safety.

If you remember, when we are in the familiarity trance, our automaticity puts us to sleep. Now, it is our fear and avoidance that hems us in or gives us cover. Our routine is a place in which we hide, so neither of us will feel anxiety or shame. However, eventually, our care becomes another prison that stifles eros and growth.

The terms of our unspoken agreement are something along these lines:

Let's not make each other uncomfortable.
Let's not ask for things that might upset the other.
Let's not act in ways that are "out of character."
Let's conceal behaviors that might be threatening to our
    partner.
Let's avoid complicated feelings and pretend that we're fine.

This kind of contract clips Cupid's wings and inhibits growth. Our tradeoff can only lead to a severe loss in our PEP and emotional engagement. Sexually, we shrink the vast ocean of each of our PEPs to the size of a small pool (see figure 5.3, "Safety Zone"). Over time, sadly, our excitement for our relationship can diminish along with our excitement for life. Since eros wants mystery, change, and also some risk, we may

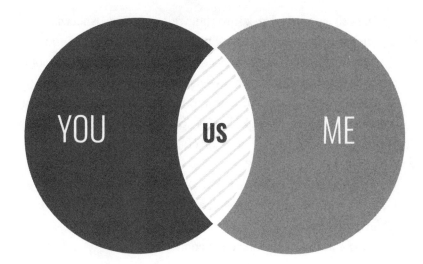

**FIGURE 5.3 SAFETY ZONE**

In the safety zone, we jettison activities that trigger shame or discomfort in either partner as our PEP shrinks considerably.

unconsciously elect for some shock treatment to wake us from our trance—a harmless flirtation, a serious affair—so that eros can roam freely again.

## TRAVELING THE NAKED PATH WITH YOUR WHOLE SELF

> The genuinely faithless one is the one who makes love to only a fraction of you and denies the rest.
> —Anaïs Nin[20]

As you can see, shrinking provides only false safety because we are hiding our real selves. A more conscious way to travel the naked path is to lean into risk. Genuine security comes when you dare to adopt a "no-mistakes" policy (i.e., no blame, no shame) when either of you risks showing different parts of yourselves. It is only by expressing rather than hiding that you keep growing and expanding together.

As was suggested above, stage 3 couples agree to support each other's self-expression, both verbally and erotically. They find ways to integrate both safety and risk into their relationship. Otherwise, like Carla, we may find ourselves engaging in covert behaviors of concealment to meet our needs for expression. Instead of securing our bond, we may end up imperiling our relationship.

As we all, consciously or unconsciously, make contracts with our partners, why not agree to make a conscious contract that is authentic, liberating, and transgressive? For starters, you can agree to:

Celebrate rather than legislate your erotic imagination.
Give the many parts of you a voice in your lovemaking.
Claim formerly exiled parts of your eroticism to transform
    shame into its opposite: deep connection.

Stage 3 couples agree to bring their whole selves to the erotic stage (the *who*) and permit themselves to partake of whichever foods they enjoy from the vast banquet eros lays out for them (the *what*). Let's now see how stage 3 couples put this agreement into practice.

## USING SHAME AS THE FUEL AND THE FIRE: PARTS PLAY

By now, we have seen that shame imprints and the safety trance can seal our erotic selves in a vacuum-packed bag. Helping couples find their authentic expression again has become a passion of mine and the impetus for an activity called parts play. It is based on the idea that we are multidimensional selves and that some parts of us long to be more integrated and fully expressed.

Often, when we think of sexual role-playing, we think of donning a French maid costume and then performing a role. Such games can be fun, but they are "outside-in." My clients tell me they want to play themselves on their erotic stage—just different ones. This inside-out approach to self-expression is much juicier than buying a Halloween costume and then matching ourselves to the outfit.

However, before we go much further, I want to talk about why we would want to engage in whole-person multimodal sex. Much of the time, sex stays in the shadows, cloaked in shame. Most of us rarely talk about sex, not with our family or friends, and often surprisingly, least of all with our partners.[21] So, while on some level we appear to be sex-saturated in the media, underneath all the bluster, many of us are more likely sex-scared. When we have sex, instead of engaging from our full self, we may take on the "safe" roles that match the cultural ideas of "hot" and "sexy" or stay locked in our "respectable" image of a grown-up.

Moreover, as we have seen, the performance trance tells us we have to be more than we are, which disconnects us only further from our innate eroticism. Stretching to be more, or contorting ourselves into something we think we should be, is oppressive. Hiding in nonthreatening and fixed roles is too. In contrast, erotic expression is emancipation from these confining scripts and roles to recover our full aliveness.

Carla was emphatic when she told me that she didn't want to go to bed with the wife, mother, and wage earner that she showed to the world. She wanted her sex life to be more like a sexy "meetup" with her other parts. After hearing similar things from other clients, I came to regard parts play as something more than just a recreational activity to break the monotony of routine sex. It is an effort to honor and integrate our diverse multidimensional selves.

If we want to stay erotically engaged, and fully alive to ourselves, then we have to find ways to bring our multiple selves into the bedroom instead of restricting sex to what Richard Schwartz calls a "predictable deployment of stereotyped parts."[22] Schwartz is the creator of Internal Family Systems, a form of psychotherapy that looks at the psyche as a family of internal parts.[23]

Before I became a therapist, I provided life planning and career services to mid-career professionals. In that role, I used an activity similar to parts play that encouraged clients to explore their unspoken dreams, aspirations, and wishes. Sometimes this activity engaged internal parts relegated to the shadows because they seemed to threaten my client's self-image or financial security.

Going inside and giving voice to those parts was liberating, exciting, and vulnerable. To many, the activity felt transgressive. It also opened them up to new and creative ways to live integrated and authentic lives.

When people successfully made a career transition or a long-sought-out lifestyle change, they were always happier. However, for a good while, many struggled to say yes to what they heard inside. Some had silenced these voices for decades, and it cost them.

The most crucial thing about this work was my inside-out approach. We used personality or interest tests only to confirm the information we gathered by journeying to their inner world and engaging with the parts that resided there. I take the same approach with erotic expression. I listen to people's fantasies and then explore which internal parts want to integrate into their partner sex. The sacred intent of parts play is to be more integrated and fully self-expressed, not to be "bigger, better, more," as the performance trance would have it.

## YOUR PASSION PYRAMID: THE FOUR FLAVORS OF EROS

I will not rest until I have told of my descent into a sensuality which was as dark, as magnificent, as wild, as my moments of mystic creation have been dazzling, ecstatic, exalted.
—Anaïs Nin[24]

If shame is the lie, the truth is that none of us would be here if not for sex. Sex is everywhere—it creates and sustains life. It also appears at all levels of the food chain. Similarly, the nourishment we receive from sex is manifold. I like to use something akin to the USDA food pyramid to illustrate four erotic "food groups" (see figure 5.4, "Passion Pyramid").

The passion pyramid helps capture the domains of experience human beings find nourishing, from the "lower" or more instinctual to the "higher" or spiritual dimensions. The pyramid is not meant to imply that one type of sex is better than another; the different layers are merely different cuisines. In other words, one kind of sex may feed the spirit, another the body. Other types of sex nourish the heart and mind.

However, if we have fixed ideas about sex, especially if they are shame-based, we may develop allergies to some of these nutrients. I

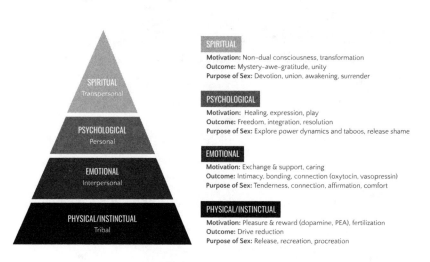

**FIGURE 5.4 PASSION PYRAMID**

Like the USDA food pyramid, eros provides different kinds of nutrients. We can nourish our body, heart, mind, or spirit through multimodal sex.

encourage you to use the passion pyramid to see if shame is preventing you from receiving the full nourishment you might require from sex. Just as we go in and out of different physical and emotional states, at different times and seasons, we may need more of one type of erotic sustenance than another.

## Physical

Let's begin with our instinctive energy, the physical gateway to eros. Our animal natures and the "reptilian" parts of our brains are what got us here and keep us here as a species. For most people, sex hormones turn on at force at puberty and compel us toward self-pleasuring and pursuing sex with another person. Throughout life, even past puberty, our physical drives can be so powerful that we might take risks that ruin hearts, or possibly override our cherished scruples.

In this way, the physical gateway is usually more about "taking" pleasure than giving. Through this lens, you may see people more as sex objects than as individuals. To follow desire in this way can feel selfish or even shameful. As a consequence, many people tend to reserve it for strangers, paid sex workers, and clandestine affairs, not for their long-term partners. Too many of us have been at the receiving end of someone else's animal motivation in a way that left us feeling used or abused. As a consequence, we may feel wary or confused about our instinctive desires.

In the context of a caring relationship, sex as "fucking" can feel very naked, even dangerous. When we notice that we have fallen into routine sex with our partner, it might be that this fear of danger has led us into the safety trance. In recognizing this, we can begin to bring our pleasure-seeking "animal" part out of hibernation. With awareness, "fucking" your partner might become one of your most naked and therefore nourishing erotic experiences together.

## Emotional

As mammals, we have not only physical but also emotional reasons for having sex. Using sex for comfort and connection is very different from pure pleasure. The bonding effect of oxytocin, which we release through sensual touch, kissing, and orgasm, deepens the sense of intimacy between people. Eros energy through the emotional portal can evoke feelings of protection, security, comfort, and generosity.

Where the physical entrance is self-focused, the emotional portal is other-focused. As a result, sex may have a sense of exchange. Since it accesses deep and heart-centered emotions, sex can have a soothing quality to it. When my client Samantha, for example, lost her father, she found making love with her partner had taken a new turn. Usually, Samantha preferred psychological forms of erotic nourishment. Sex now brought a quality of deep connection that unexpectedly reassured her that she was "not alone."

A common stereotype is that men approach sex primarily through the animal gateway. According to Terrence Real, a family therapist who specializes in men's issues, "The only two emotions allowed men under patriarchy are anger and lust. Some men filter all of their emotional needs and expression into sex; they wear their hearts on their genitals."[25]

The emotional gate is not without risks, however. When sex is a means of expressing a heart-centered connection, the emotional gateway can feel as naked and as vulnerable as showing our animal side to our partner. That is why shame and the safety trance can show up here too. If it feels risky to "give our heart" to our partner when we have sex, we may be mesmerized by an overarching need for safety. It can also be the case that losing sexual interest in our partner is a way of protecting ourselves from being hurt. We might avoid exposing what we consider to be our shameful flaws by avoiding this portal altogether.

## Psychological

Our psychological motivations for sex are self-expression, healing, and play. Esther Perel says, "Animals have sex; eroticism is exclusively human. It is sexuality transformed by the imagination."[26] Through the psychological gate, we may set up elaborate scenarios to try on new roles, ages, and genders, or to heal early wounds. Thus, this channel includes the nourishment of role-playing and kink.

Unfortunately, even the most fun loving and adventurous of us become contained when we believe that there is too much at stake to be daring. However, keeping our all-important relationship on an even, if not routine, keel, can snuff out our creativity.

It might surprise you to hear that 36 percent of adults in the United States use masks, blindfolds, and bondage tools during sex. Is this behavior pathological? Well, despite whatever assumptions we might make about bondage, flogging, and dungeons, the data suggests otherwise. People who are into the BDSM (bondage and discipline, dominance and submission, sadomasochism) "lifestyle" frequently score better on measurements of anxiety, depression, and PTSD than the rest of the population.[27]

So, does this mean we should run out and try it? The kind of sex we enjoy is partly hardwired, and, like other tastes, partly acquired. However, our attitudes toward various sexual activities have a lot to do with the zeitgeist—what's fashionable and accepted by our culture today. While the so-called Grey Trend (named after the success of *Fifty Shades of Grey*) is popular now, it is certainly not for everyone.[28] So, while you may be ready to explore your kinky side, your partner may cringe at the thought, or vice-versa. We don't have to partake in anything we have no taste for, nor do we have to hide our favorite flavors out of shame.

## Spiritual

When eros energy moves through the spiritual gateway, many people believe it offers an experience of communion with the divine, life, and possibly the entire universe. Experiences of altered and ecstatic states of transcendence are associated with the spiritual gateway. People who source nourishment here report a sense of oneness with all of nature, a melding wherein the ego dissolves and "the living spirit can be felt and shared in its pure form."[29]

Of course, it is easy for shame and the safety trance to stand in the way of these transpersonal delights as well. We may have created a false dichotomy between sex and spirit, believing the body is impure or that sex is too "base." However, many people that I have worked with are hugely relieved to discover that sex and spirituality make extraordinary bedmates and that they can feed both aspects of themselves at the same time.

Having a sense of the many flavors and motivations for sex can expand your creative expression enormously. Moreover, each of your parts has particular culinary preferences, and these may reflect different needs that are prevailing at different times. For example, you might have an internal part that enjoys transpersonal sex while also at other times another part of you that prefers to partake of sex as emotional food. You might have an internal part named "Witchy Dom" that likes food from the psychological part of the banquet and a "Randy Rhino" part that enjoys the animal food group.

As a couple, I encourage you to explore whether your parts usually crave the same or different foods through sex. Do you have enough foods that your parts both enjoy that you can live on a shared meal plan? If not, make sure each of them gets at least some of what they crave occasionally. If their appetites are different, you have to decide how to eat together. Can you eat separate things at the same meal? Many couples have different motivations for sex and make out just fine. For example, one of you might be looking for a release and the other for play. If you both get at least a tad of what you are after, then you are likely to be satisfied.

Unfortunately, many stage 2 couples, often without ever verbally agreeing on it, come to rely primarily on one of these food groups. The pyramid shows there are different kinds of nourishment we can get from sex. Being bored with your sexual diet is an opportunity to bring different parts of you forward and also to explore the type of sexual cuisine each of you is seeking. Moving out of your erotic home base can certainly feel naked with your long-term partner, but it can also be potentially thrilling for the parts that have a diverse erotic palate.

## DIFFERENT STROKES: WHEN ONE PERSON'S PASSION IS ANOTHER PERSON'S POISON

As we have seen, on the naked path erotic expression happens in two dimensions: what we do, or the "what" of our sexual experience (the four basic food groups), and "who" we are when we enjoy them (our various internal erotic parts). By exploring your fantasies, you can find out which food groups appeal to your parts. You can then explore what kinds of meals you might want to cook and with which ingredients.

As we explore the passion pyramid together, we may find that our partner wants to eat something that we have trouble swallowing. While we often focus on the titillating aspects of sex, many sexual activities also turn us off. In Buddhism, pushing away things that frighten, trigger, or repulse us is considered to be a principal cause of our suffering. Aversion is thus deemed to be a "poison" because it closes us off to life.[30]

Aversion is also at the center of the safety trance, for when we privilege security over risk, we banish from the bedroom anything that makes us uncomfortable. Areas of the body can become off-limits, as are times of day, specific activities, and even words that might trigger a shame response. Through this process of elimination, David Schnarch claims that most couples subsist on sexual "leftovers."[31]

The antidote to aversion is not avoidance or hiding but to include, embrace—even love—what we fear. Does this mean we have to say yes to everything our partner desires? Not at all. Giving all of our parts a voice in our relationship means we provide as much consideration to the parts that say no, as the parts that say yes. However, we can open to our partner's wishes by seeing what we can discover about our aversive reaction through mindful self-study. Doing so is the antidote to the poison of aversion and the *caring* side of our contract.

When sex becomes a portal for knowing ourselves, we lose our fear of touching into feelings of discomfort because we have the means to encounter them, mindfully, as an erotic team. We may discover something that allows us to expand erotically, but this is not always the goal.

It is worth repeating that there are often good reasons for setting limits and boundaries. We may have a genuine allergy to something. The problem is not that we have boundaries, but how we erect them. Our protective strategies are often unconscious and disconnecting. They wall us off from the deeper and more vulnerable parts of ourselves. Consequently, these parts remain mysterious and charged, like a live volcano. When we bring loving-kindness toward something we want to push away, our aversions can bring us closer to our partner and ourselves. Thus, exploring our reactions as a mindful team is an essential aspect of the naked path to re-enchantment.

## CONSCIOUS PARTS PLAY AND PLAYLISTS

The erotic creativity of eros, as we have seen, relies on imagination and at times, fantasy.

All of us have a stock "playlist" of erotic motifs that arouse us. We tend to play out these motifs, privately, in our imagination. However, at stage 3, we may take our nakedness to another level by giving our partner a private screening. We can also go further by bringing ourselves out from the shadows of shame and into the "us" zone of the Venn diagram by enjoying these pleasures with our partner. In so doing, erotic expression leads to erotic expansion (see figure 5.5, "Erotic Expansion").

In our retreats, we guide people through a silent mindful replay of their typical repertoire: What do you and your partner do when you have sex? In other words, "What's your typical meal?" Then each names the parts of themselves that play together on their erotic stage with their partner. Afterward, we do a second exercise where we have them go into an arousal fantasy, something they might use to get off when they

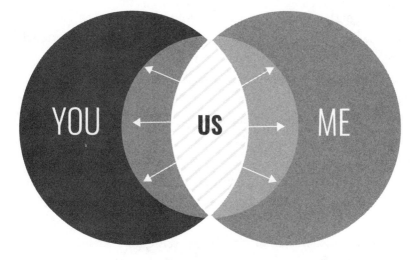

**FIGURE 5.5 EROTIC EXPANSION**

At stage 3, we expand our safety zone by bringing our multidimensional selves and their appetites out from the shadows and into the "us" zone.

masturbate. From this exercise, we can identify which parts want expression and also where on the pyramid these parts want to play. It is by combining various parts and palettes that we experience whole-person multimodal sex.

Of course, many people are embarrassed and ashamed of their fantasies. Take a moment to notice what happens when you imagine doing this activity. Feel around for any shame reactions. Imagine your partner could see clear into you; including the private scenarios that turn you on when you pleasure yourself. What other parts would they see in you besides the ones that play together in your safety zone? Shame lives in this secret hiding spot. Don't turn the lights on just yet; explore the shadows for a while.

## FANTASY AND FOOD GROUPS

Fantasy allows us to utilize shame in extraordinary, creative ways. If you allow yourself this privilege, you triumph over shame.

—Joy Davidson[32]

Investigating fantasy scenarios can illuminate fears and self-judgments. As Carla and I ran through this exercise, she realized that she struggles to reconcile her "dark" fantasies with her identity as a "feminist" and "humanitarian." Her ambivalence is understandable, given that Carla is working on a campaign to end domestic violence. "How can I possibly enjoy being overpowered at night?" she asks, looking horrified. Carla is unaware that power lies not in any particular act, but with the person who has the control.

I explain that in her fantasies, Carla is the director, screenwriter, casting agent, and actor, which means she can always yell, "Cut!" For just this reason, enacting fantasies within the safe container of a committed, consensual relationship is an entirely different context than being the victim of another person's misuse of power. Carla looks relieved, particularly when I add that fantasies rarely line up with our values or politics. Just as our night dreams can be disturbing so too can our "day" dreams. While a part of us gets excited, another part looks on aghast.

Some years back, the wife of a couple that attended my Passion and Presence retreat grabbed me on a break and in a conspiratorial tone said, "My fantasies disturb me, and I'd like to talk to you about it." She looked to see if anyone, particularly her husband, was in earshot before continuing. "Well, when I masturbate, I always imagine a crowd of men poking me with sticks and jeering me." "Um-hum," I uttered, waiting for her to continue. She looked dumbfounded. "Well, there's something wrong with that, isn't there? Why would I want to be treated that way? Do I think that little of myself?"

"What part of the fantasy is the peak point of arousal?" I asked, using a technique developed by Jack Morin.[33] She got mindful and then said, "When they say the phrase 'Show me what you've got,' in a way that feels like both a demand and a dare." "Hear the phrase inside, and mindfully study what happens inside of you at that moment?" I suggested. "Well, it's like all the restraints come down, and I can be truly sexually free. I know that whatever I do, however whorish I act, I will get applause."

"So, do you feel small and disempowered in the fantasy?" I asked, already knowing the answer. "No, I feel like the most powerful woman on earth, and like my most wicked desires will be fully received." After a long pause, she slapped my knee and said, "Thanks. I'm ready to go back inside."

If we were doing parts play, we would come up with a name for this part, like "Saucy Wench." We would find out what kind of context would support the part's expression (a barn, outdoors, standing, bright light, darkness). Would it need props? Sticks, perhaps? What tone of voice would her husband use when saying, "Show me what you've got!" Since the fantasy involves the motifs of humiliation and power, she is sourcing nourishment from the psychological food group. We might mindfully explore any barriers or concerns she or her husband have about this kind of play.

By using this approach, Carla realized she was longing for more "edge." The routine of Miguel bringing her to orgasm through oral sex and then entering her for a minute or two was not only staid and predictable but also too tame. It lacked the passion she played out in images of being taken. In other words, she wanted more animal energy in their encounters.

Miguel, in turn, realized that he was starved for spiritual nourishment. Early in their relationship, Miguel suggested they light candles and look into each other's eyes before making love. Carla raised an eyebrow and said, "Are you going New Age-y on me now?" Miguel felt ridiculed and decided to stick to the program in the future. Though in his private fantasies, he enjoys being with women who are interested in going slow and honoring the connection between them.

Like many couples, neither Carla nor Miguel talked about that incident or their dulling implicit contract. They used the children and their busy schedules to excuse their lack of creativity in bed. By talking openly and accepting their different preferences, they were able to codesign a scenario that combined the "sacred" and "animal."

To get started, Miguel took a few minutes in mindfulness and felt into his "devotional" energy, as he now openly called it. Mindfulness helps us locate our many parts because it turns us back inside. As we quiet the noise in our system, we become more sensitive. We can listen for who's in there, who wants to speak, and how.

As Miguel let fantasy images come into his mind, he saw his head between Carla's breasts and was smelling her skin. Carla recoiled upon hearing this, and her hands instinctively went to cover her breasts. As mentioned, an automatic impulse to retract, constrict, or avert our gaze may be indicators of shame.

Carla was now quite taken with the practice of mindful self-study and wondered what she might learn about her reaction. She turned her attention inward and studied her hands. Carla noticed that she felt very exposed and that some anger was welling up too. By staying with her present experience in an open and exploratory way, Carla started to understand her aversive response to Miguel's image.

She recalls growing breasts before her friends did and getting unwanted attention not only from the boys at school but also from her friends' fathers. The thought of Miguel "peering" at her breasts frankly "creeped her out." We wondered together if this might be an opportunity to plant a heart as the pain of her young self was here.

Carla said she wished she had been invisible back then, that she could have hidden. Miguel asked if she wanted him to sit in front of her with his back to her. That way, no one, including himself, would be able to see her. She liked that idea very much. Once Miguel repositioned himself, Carla let out a deep sigh. She connected with a younger part of her that never had a chance to enjoy her breasts; they were always a source of fear and humiliation.

After another ten minutes of being together this way, they came up with a creative way to plant hearts at home. Carla wanted to reconnect to her breasts appreciatively and to honor her shyness. She had the image of sitting across from Miguel and engaging in a game of "tit-and-seek." She laughed freely at the thought. She explained that she was imagining herself wearing a white towel and flashing him every few seconds. The idea of being in charge of what he could see was enticing to another part she called the "Coy Fox." Coy Fox is the part that longs for more seduction between her and Miguel, she explained, "but she doesn't want to ask for it."

Carla also enjoyed imagining spreading her legs when she opened the towel to tease Miguel. Doing this would allow Carla to feel the raw animal energy she had been hungering for these many years. Miguel said he was up for all of this and was getting hot just hearing about the intended activity. He asked if they could light candles and put flowers in the room to create the kind of space he imagined in his "erotic arts temple" fantasy. She agreed.

The couple was in good spirits when they left arm in arm and hopeful about finally having the kind of sex together that they had been having in their imaginations. Before leaving, they decided to arrange a weekend playdate for the kids and to have one for themselves at the same time.

## BEYOND OUR CREATIVE DIFFERENCES: USING A MULTIMODAL APPROACH

Sometimes couples' parts trigger each other in ways that lead to an impasse as we saw with Eric and Max in chapter 3. Richard Schwartz, from whom I learned a lot about working with internal parts, describes a couple he worked with where the husband, Mark, developed a hypersexual part called "the Stud" to overcome shame for having large nipples as a teenager.[34] His partner Stacey also carried shame from an early childhood incident in which her father's energy uncomfortably changed when he was bathing her. Both Mark and Stacy had exiled the younger internal parts that were carrying shame and in Stacey's case, fear. As a result, Stacey had developed a part she called "the Prude."

Not surprisingly, each time the Stud approached Stacey for sex, the Prude automatically recoiled, which, in turn, created more shame for Mark. However, once they both understood the source of these protector parts they could implement a "no child left behind" policy. For as Schwartz explains, these younger exiled parts (what I call the protected) contain not just hurt and shame, but also "give us our capacity for joy, love, passion, creativity, imagination, playfulness, and sheer zest for life."[35]

By now, you can see that on the naked path, we use everything that occurs inside of us to become self-aware and also to expand our PEP. At stage 3, our commitment to erotic expression compels us to research how we may be containing our own impulses or stifling our partner's self-expression. In such instances, we use mindful coinvestigation to study the reasons for this. For example, partner A might make a gesture, facial expression, or statement that captures the energy of a challenging part for partner B. In response, partner B takes time to get mindful and then researches and shares their reactions to the trigger.

When one of *our* internal parts is restraining another *inner* part, it is useful to see what might happen if it wasn't doing that. As an example, we may have a "Party Pooper" part that finds the activities that appeal to a "Bonobo" part disgusting. Through mindful self-study, we may discover that the Party Pooper is judging Bonobo to protect it from being humiliated.

We never want to override our well-intended protectors. Doing so creates a power struggle within ourselves, and our sexual engagement will be half-hearted at best. However, if we explore the wound behind the protector, we may discover an opportunity to plant a heart as Miguel did with Carla, and Carla did with herself. Again, using the erotic portal for healing and growth is the essence of the naked path.

Quite a few of the couples who attend our retreats are initially embarrassed, even intimidated, by parts play. However, they also delight in the freedom to act "out of character." Carla and Miguel were able to easily connect their erotic parts through movement. During a "parts dance" at our retreat, Carla came up to me and remarked, "I'm no longer bored!" Now she and Miguel have in-home dances often. They take turns curating an evocative playlist and move, seduce, and touch the other in ways that allow their parts to connect without words.

Another couple, Jay and Nina, happened upon a fun and naughty game that they call "Not Tonight Dear." When Jay is too tired for sex, with consent, Nina calls on an internal part she named the "Sexy Massage Therapist," and takes things "into her own hands." Alternatively (with permission), one of Jay's parts, called "the Hunter," might say to a tired Nina, "You don't have to enjoy it. I'll use you." As Jay becomes aroused, Nina's sleepiness often leaves and "Frisky Frieda" wakes up to get in on the action.

When Stacey and Mark overcame their impasse, they were able to bring in lots of different parts to their lovemaking. "Stacey reported that she'd suddenly find herself moving in ways she'd never moved before and saying words she'd never said, and all the different parts seemed to find great joy in finally expressing themselves as openly and physically as they wanted."[36]

Carla and Miguel had a similar experience. Initially, they set up a scenario that enabled Carla to feel a sense of seduction and danger. Miguel set up a temple space for his "Goddess Worshipper." However, once they were a few scenes in, other parts emerged that added surprise and delight to their love-making so that it felt exciting and new.

## WHY PARTAKE IN WHOLE-PERSON SEX?

Today, sexual satisfaction has become a mandate in long-term relationships. That wasn't always the case. At the same time, more couples are taking what has become the "realistic view." They cite the statistic that half of us will stray before we get to the "'til death do us part" mark, particularly with our longer lifespans. Now, more than ever, our relationship container needs to be elastic, they say, if we have a chance of lasting nearly that long. It is for this reason that more and more people see consensual non-monogamy as a valid option.

As a couple, I encourage you to discuss how you feel about "outside attractions" as well as porn, flirting, and live and cyber sexual encounters with others. At what point does it cross the line and become cheating? There are no right and wrong answers here; these are questions you will want to explore together as you discuss the topic of erotic expression and your relational contract.[37] However, as you have seen, on the naked path being exclusive does not have to come at a cost to erotic expression. As Ian Kerner, a sex and relationships expert, says, "We don't need a variety of sexual partners to spice up our sex lives; we just need to update the menu more regularly and offer a more inventive selection of daily specials."[38]

As presented here, parts play can be an exciting and liberating "special." You can make love to and as "other people" without opening your relationship or cheating. In sharing his sexual experience of meeting without fixed roles, the essayist and cultural critic Michael Ventura writes, "To see suddenly, upon someone long loved, a face you've never seen is unnerving, and some part of you wants to say, 'Honey, put your mask back on,' while some other part of you wants to say, 'Who are you? And how do I get to know you better?'"[39]

## DARING TO BE FULLY ALIVE

"Good Knight, where are you going?" asks the queen to a knight played by the actor George Clooney. The actor is stepping out of the movie screen and into the theater. Because this is a commercial, he then makes his way to a coffee store.[40] If your erotic part walked off the screen of your intimate theater, what would it be wearing? (Knight regalia, a spacesuit, or something slinky?) How would it speak? Where would you find it hanging out? In the commercial above, Peter Gabriel is singing "Solsbury Hill."[41] What soundtrack would your character want to come fully alive?

Each of these questions pertains to context. What context will help you drop into parts play more fully, without feeling self-conscious or like you are manufacturing a part? With this inside-out approach to exploring the characters in their inner worlds, most couples feel more intimate and connected, as well as more freely expressed.

Not uncommonly, however, people tell me that they don't fantasize at all, and that's okay too. I have come to learn that many have images in their mind of the kind of sex they find arousing, but their scenario is more PG than X-rated. While we typically think the X-rated stuff is racy, for some of the people that I work with, having eyes-open sex is far more daring than being tied up. Thus, erotic expression is integrating whichever parts we have exiled to the shadows, including soft, tender, and possibly gender-fluid parts.

One way we put eros in a box is when we put the kibosh on our transgressive or gender nonconforming fantasies because they scare or repel us. Eros is a fervent gender bender. Eros energy shamelessly flows through all of the erotic food groups and shape-shifts from one moment to the next. The same energy flows through us in myriad ways. Iasenza, the feminist psychoanalyst mentioned earlier, calls this expanded erotic space "queer space," because sexual thoughts, desires, behaviors, attractions, and sensations are fluid and multidimensional. Embracing all of our sexual dimensions is how we triumph over shame and reclaim our sovereign erotic power.

## MINDFUL ACTIVITIES AND NAKED REFLECTIONS

. . . . . . . . . . . . . . . . . . . . . . . . . . . . . . . . . . . . . . . . . . . . . . . . . . . . . . . . . . . . . . .

## Experiencing the Creative Potential of Parts Play

. . . . . . . . . . . . . . . . . . . . . . . . . . . . . . . . . . . . . . . . . . . . . . . . . . . . . . . . . . . . . . .

Parts play has many levels. We may choose to embody the part and speak and move under its sway in a sexual or nonsexual context. We might go further and use props, attire, music, and other features in the environment to create a context to support the part's expression. Alternatively, we may engage in an inside-out version of role-playing, where we set up a scenario in which both partner's parts interact in some way.

Here you will explore and process your fantasies without being sexual (except for the last step). As a couple, you can decide how far you want to go. It's fine to do each step during separate meetings. Because you will be doing the first two activities individually, you can do those at different times. If you choose this option, be sure each of you takes notes to refer to later.

### *Exploring Your Erotic Imagination (15–20 minutes)*
### Mindful Self-Study

Do 5 minutes of mindfulness. Then, bring to mind a sexual fantasy that you use to arouse yourself. If none come to mind, then create an ideal imaginary sexual encounter. Run through the fantasy and let yourself enjoy it. Now, go through the scenario a second time as an observer. The intention is to gather information about the specifics of the fantasy and what you find arousing.

How do you get to be in this fantasy (passive, in charge, demanding, coy, playful, daring)? What do you wear? What kinds of things do you say and do? Look for details. Where does this take place? Who else is there? What are they doing, and how do they treat you?

Among other aspects, you may want to explore the following:

Are you giving or receiving?
Is there a big seduction or do you go for it right away?
What words, if any, are being exchanged?
What kind of sex are you having?
What do you get to experience in the fantasy that you don't with your partner?

## Exploring Barriers to Sharing (10 minutes)
### Mindful Self-Study

Do a few minutes of mindfulness meditation. Then, imagine sharing your fantasy with your partner. What happens automatically? Notice any body sensations, feelings, impulses, or images that arise when you consider letting your partner see this aspect of you. What happens in your energy? Do you speed up, flatten out, tense, become teary, anxious, or frozen when you imagine sharing your wish? Be curious about what kind of state starts to develop. Let the emotional response tell you about itself.

Try to stay close to your feelings. See if you can discover something previously unknown to you about how you inhibit your aliveness or censor yourself. What assumptions do you carry about how your partner will react if you tell them your fantasy? What happens when you believe this reaction to be real? How does this contribute to hiding? How might the safety trance be inhibiting you from expressing this part? Are you afraid of triggering your partner, or is your shame holding you back in some way?

Do the remaining activities together as a couple.

## Sharing Barriers to Expression with Your Partner
(About 10 minutes per person, however, take all the time you need. Don't rush this step.)

Decide who will go first or whether you will only go one round in this session. Partner A shares discoveries from the exploring barriers activity. Don't share the content of your fantasy yet. Instead, what do you think could happen, or go wrong if you share your imagination (whether this is realistic or not)? Tell your partner the assumptions you carry about how they will react. Practice the three R's and reveal your hidden vulnerability about letting your partner see this part of you. Discuss what you might need to come out of hiding.

### Sharing a Piece of the Fantasy (15 minutes or more, per person)

Make sure you have a private place in which to speak that is also free of interruptions. Decide ahead of time if each of you will have a chance to share, or if you will focus on only one of you for this particular session. Also, only do this activity when you are both in good states separately and as a couple.

The first thing to remember is that sharing our desires is more important than doing the desired activity. Second, you want to foster a sense of compassionate teamwork throughout this process. Be alert for any indicators of shame and go slow in such instances.

To begin with, as the *sharer*, start with something positive, such as what you appreciate about your partner. Then share something about your fantasy and what makes it appealing. A mindful approach involves peeling back the surface request to reveal the *underlying intrigue*. Allow your curiosity to be present throughout the exchange.

As the *listener*, the *caring* part of your contract is a willingness to be curious when your partner expresses a desire or fantasy. They are daring to be vulnerable by sharing their private world with you. You might ask questions such as, "How is it to speak about your desire?" "What do you imagine you will experience that will be exciting?"

As a *listener*, you will also want to observe your habits and tendencies regarding how you listen and regulate yourself to stay curious and compassionate. If something you hear triggers an unpleasant internal reaction, your commitment is to stop, study, and share. That is, pause, and engage in mindful self-study. Then report on what you have learned from doing so.

If things get too heated, and your protectors are showing up, take a time-out. However, agree that during the break, you will be working with your state and seeing what you are protecting. Use the PREP process you learned in chapter 3 if you need "emergency roadside assistance."

If possible, focus on the exchange as an opportunity to know your partner more intimately, not to rush into any action.

### Naming the Part and Its Preferences (20 minutes or more, per person)

After one of you has shared your fantasy, take time together to get to know the part that is active in the fantasy. Imagine you have invited it to visit you both for tea. See this part as another person in the room with you. How does this part behave in your presence? Is it dominant/submissive, flirty, teasing, nurturing, naughty, controlling, innocent, rejecting, admiring? What is it wearing? How does it speak? Stay curious and nonjudging as you try to get to know this part. Remember, you have lots of internal parts. Undoubtedly, some of them want different things and may even judge this part's appetites or persona.

Now, come up with a name for this part. After you have named the part identify the area on the passion pyramid that seems to be this part's playground.

You can stay with one partner's exploration for the session or switch directions and go through the steps again for the other partner. After both of you have completed this activity, spend time exploring how each partner's parts get along. How do they feel toward one another? Do they find each other sexy or do they have an aversive reaction to the other? If the latter is the case, see if you can find another internal part to play with together if you choose to do the remaining activities.

### Nonsexual Parts Play (set a timer to limit the activity or keep it open-ended)

Each of you will select a part to play with for a period outside of the bedroom. Allow that part to have "center stage" in your interaction and being in the world. Dress in a way that expresses this part. It is okay to feel self-conscious but don't take it too seriously. This activity is "play" time, a time of experimentation, and improvisation. Try to avoid putting any performance pressure on yourself or your partner to get it "right," or "perfect." Be lighthearted together as you both relate to each other in character in a nonsexual context. Let the parts go out to dinner, sing and dance, or take a walk together. Let them speak and interact verbally and nonverbally. Open your playfulness and act out your parts. Later, share what that was like for each of you.

### Engaging in Sexual Parts Play

Should you decide to "go all the way," you can bring these parts to bed with you. You can engage in unscripted erotic play, or you can first codesign a scenario for how these parts would relate in a sexual context. Take this activity only as far as you want to go.

If you decide to create a scenario, first pretend you are directing a scene from a play. Describe the characters and their connection to each other. What is the context of the interaction? Where are they, what would be bringing them together? Do they need any props, or music to feel more expressed? Be as specific as you can be to "set the stage."

Once you start the activity, pause periodically to explore barriers and feelings evoked by parts play mindfully. The intention is not to have a fantastic experience but rather to experiment together. Be sure to explore as a team rather than trying to reach the goal of an excellent encounter. After the activity, spend a few minutes nakedly sharing observations, feelings, and reactions.

Remember, you can use your stop signal any time during the exercise. If you find that your anxiety goes beyond a four on a ten-point scale, stop. Take time to de-role. Say your real name, put on something comforting and familiar to your partner, and lie on your sides, face-to-face, looking at one another until you feel settled.

. . . . . . . . . . . . . . . . . . . . . . . . . . . . . . . . . . . . . . . . . . . . . . . . . . . . . . . . . . . . . . . . .

## Naked Reflections
. . . . . . . . . . . . . . . . . . . . . . . . . . . . . . . . . . . . . . . . . . . . . . . . . . . . . . . . . . . . . . . . .

What did you learn about yourself from doing this activity, including your limits? How was it to interact sexually with your different parts?

What new experiences were you able to open up to, and which impulses did you inhibit during the encounter? How can parts play help you overcome shame? What do you want to do differently next time?

# 6.

## EROTIC ATTUNEMENT

### Dancing with Eros from the Inside Out

Open yourself to the Tao, then trust your natural responses; and everything will fall into place.
—LAO TZU, *TAO TE CHING*[1]

I am sitting with Owen and Seth, a fun-loving mid-thirties couple that
identifies as "monogamish." For them, that means they can each have
sex with other people while traveling for business, as long as there are
no emotional ties. The couple occasionally brings a third person into
their bed, which they say happens maybe once or twice a year. Alone,
at home, however, both lament that their erotic life has become utterly
predictable.

Seth takes a few minutes to rough out one of the three fantasy scenarios they rely on to get off together. In this scene, nineteen-year-old
Owen has never been with a man. Seth is Owen's twenty-three-year-old
brother's friend and is visiting at their house. When Owen's brother
goes to the grocery store for beer, Seth rubs up against Owen and acts
as if it was an accident. He then starts asking Owen questions to keep
him engaged. Eventually, he pushes things a bit further, proceeding
from touching his genitals to oral sex, and so on. Of course, all of this
has to happen before Owen's brother comes home.

While the scenario contains all of the elements that the erotic mind finds arousing—risk, the forbidden, obstacle, and chase[2]—the mystery left this weathered fantasy years ago. When our fun and sexy "specials" become standard fare, they eventually lose their flavor. Moreover, while parts play is a way to liberate our repressed parts, reenacting a set scenario can also be a place to hide from one another. It's like a racy version of the safety trance.

Unfortunately, many of us latch onto what was once (or promises to be) a fail-proof recipe for hot sex, only to find ourselves starved for eros. For this reason, it is good to heed the words of Peggy Kleinplatz, who puts it plainly: "There is nothing that kills desire faster than the pursuit of what works, relentlessly."[3]

In contrast, stage 3 couples stay enchanted erotically by opening to what each moment calls forward in themselves and their partner. Without an agenda or fixed plan in mind, they meet what's here—in this moment—and respond accordingly. Rather than playing roles to *make* things erotic, you too can learn how to *attune* to the eros energy unfolding between you both, and allow this to lead you to erotic pleasures. I call this ability "erotic attunement"; it is an essential skill of being present to passion.

Erotic attunement is like the art of improvisation. For example, contact improvisation is a dance form that requires the letting go of a sense of "willfulness" so that the "natural flow of movement" can be expressed. In this way, the dancing itself facilitates the fine-tuning of the senses, so the "ability to listen and respond to what is happening in the moment" is awakened.[4]

Similarly, erotic attunement helps you both *find* and *express* the natural flow of eros moving through and between you. By attuning to eros, you locate your passion and presence, which leads to your pleasure. It is for this reason that many couples come to our retreats hoping to get what we are covering in this chapter right off the bat. However, without the scaffolding we have been building and the skills to work with triggers, in particular, it is easy to give up the dance or default back to our numbing routines.

It is only fair to tell you that this chapter doesn't teach fancy moves or specific pleasuring techniques. Many books on sexual enrichment teach you how to be "better" at sex as if, like tennis, you can improve your game with a better forehand. On the naked path we don't need an instruction manual because we align with life moving through us.

When we rely on erotic attunement and connect to ourselves in this moment, we find we know what to do. Here it is also important to shed the judge's cap and cultivate a spirit of exploration and play. In fact, to find our full-bodied PEP we need to recover the sense that there are infinite paths we might take each time we make love.

To test this claim, you can try connecting to the infinite possibilities available in this moment to move and stretch your body. Take a few minutes and try this right now:

Sense your body, front to back, top and bottom, left and right. Take a full minute to do this. As you check in with yourself, find some way your body might like to move. Try to erase images of stretches you've learned in fitness classes and listen to your body. Tune into any impulses to bend, twist, reach, shake, or fold up in familiar or habitual ways. Be open to new directions and inspirations. It might be as simple as first stretching your left arm instead of your right arm. If it feels good, keep going, and enjoy it. Otherwise, adjust to make it better and try again. Take another couple of minutes to enjoy following your internal guidance.

For most of us, trusting this internal guide or what in body psychotherapy is called our felt sense[5] is easier said than done. Feelings of shame, the daze of trances, and the pull of hidden factors disconnect us from our eros energy regularly. It is for this very reason that every chapter until now has addressed one or more barriers to sexual vitality. As we have seen, these barriers lock us into outdated sexual scripts and what I call *outside-in* pathways to pleasure. The dance of sex becomes no longer an improvisation but more a polished routine.

Children are masters of improvisation—when music comes on they often move and sway without any self-consciousness, seemingly unconcerned with getting it "right." Their body just knows what to do without a single dance lesson. They move from the *inside-out*. As adults, we have barriers, but we can indeed find such a state again if we tap our animating force.

## RECOVERING OUR "ELEMENTAL WILD SPIRIT"

> The creative person always walks two steps into the darkness.
> That's where you discover "other things," the things that defy
> description.
> —Benny Golson, jazz musician and composer[6]

"We are vessels for the life force." These are the words that struck me so powerfully as I listened to Tara Brach (a psychologist, author, and founder of the Insight Meditation Community in Washington, DC) speak at a large convention for psychotherapists. This was not the first time I had heard such an idea, but something this time struck me in a new way. There was an implication that I hadn't quite appreciated before: I was the carrier of something precious, and therefore my whole being, including my body, was a container of an energetic, life-giving power.

Soon after, I began to contemplate how this life-force energy doesn't belong to us. It comes through us—in fact, we are "the sons and daughters of Life's longing for itself," as Kahlil Gibran put it.[7] Of course, Freud spoke of libido as psychic energy or the life instinct that compels us to have sex. Modern-day sexologists as well as Tantra and Taoist sexuality practitioners also refer to eros energy.

However, until I heard the word *vessel*, I was unable to shake my aversion to the mechanical "tension and release" model that the word *energy* conjured, and that often framed traditional body psychotherapy. Now I felt differently. I was no longer concerned with what animates us, but what I could do to help my clients tune into *themselves* to connect to this universal turn-on.

When I approached eros in this way, I soon realized that it has proclivities independent of ours. Sexual enrichment interventions that emphasize outside-in maneuvers and techniques rely on the application of a certain level of willfulness to direct sexual "energy." In contrast, I began to appreciate that an inside-out approach saw "good

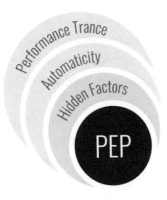

FIGURE 6.1 CHAPTER 6 PEP BARRIERS

sex" as more about sensing and responding to the eros energy in an organic, improvisational way; that is, rather than trying to direct eros, we must learn to follow it. As a result, *being present* is what enlivens passion and pleasure.

Erotic attunement connects us to ourselves and to eros energy in the pursuit of sexual pleasure. If we can imagine ourselves as a vessel for eros, we might feel less shame around expressing our fundamental aliveness in whole-body ways. We might also experience less performance pressure and goal orientation. Eros energy is the music, and we are the dancer animated by the music within.

Reconnecting to—or discovering—this ability to tune into the animating force of our erotic energy is entirely possible. However, for most people, it usually takes some practice, since many of us have become wedded to the performance mind-set. You may recall that a performance mind-set is fused with the cultural imperative to excel at everything we do, including sex.

Mindful sex, like mindfulness practice, is not goal focused; it is present focused. Therefore, on the naked path, we must be aware of and willing to drop our performance mind-set and the habits it leads to when it comes to sex. We can no more attain "perfect" sex than "perfect" meditation. To the contrary, mindful sex is allowing a far-from-perfect performance.

K. Anders Ericsson, a professor at the University of Florida, tells a story about how competitive ice skaters develop mastery but look awful in the process—with lessons we can apply in our approach to sex. In practice sessions, these skaters look terrible because they are always trying something new. In contrast, skaters that perform professionally but are not training for competition, look polished because they repeat the same routines over and over.

Ericsson stresses that mastery is more than a result of time and repetition: we do not become experts by repeating something for 10,000 hours.[8] Repetition leads to *automaticity* rather than excellence in skaters, as well as musicians, cardiologists, and any other group. The research suggests that we become masterful only by going to our edge and meeting uncertainty, not by repeating the same moves each time.[9]

Unfortunately, like professional skaters, many of us focus on how we look, trying to get our moves just right when we have sex. We stay within tight lines, safeguarding ourselves from appearing foolish or stepping on each other's toes. This form of "safe sex" only deadens eros. We end up exiling the wild, messy, and exploratory parts of ourselves that help us discover "other things."

As Welwood says, we can fully appreciate the "transformative quality" of sex, only when "we connect with our elemental wild spirit, which is forever unfathomable to the rational mind."[10] From the perspective of eros, good lovers do best when they do less thinking and planning about sex, and let their bodies move in response to the energy unfolding between them. In this "wild" approach, everything, including "mistakes," becomes part of the dance.

Sadly, it is all too easy to be in our heads about what great sex should look like, or used to look like, or to struggle with ideas that create anxiety around performance. However, if we approach sex through our template of a "good performance," we are at risk of turning into the pretty looking skaters who do the same routine over and over.

While humans, as living systems, rely on internal models as guideposts,[11] mindful sex involves going into the dark without the expectation—and the pressure—of perfect performance. We have to *feel into* our eros energy and be present enough to notice signals from our partner that tell us to move faster or slower, lick or pinch.

Improvisation is a practice in itself. We can be wildly experimental only if we agree there are no mistakes. In this approach, nothing is a problem, and nothing is to be rejected as "wrong." For example, I once took a salsa workshop with an instructor who demonstrated the art of "falling." Instead of sloughing off the potentially embarrassing moment that can happen to any salsa dancer, she showed us how to incorporate it into the dance itself. The "mistake" of falling became hot, graceful, and connecting.

Improv artists do the same thing, especially when working with another person or in a group. They always join with what is there in the moment and then, take it a step further. Instead of digging in, or working at cross-purposes with others, they stay light on their feet. They move in response to what is emerging in the now.

Stage 3 couples also assume this readiness to "join with" each other. With erotic attunement, they stay in touch with eros energy and allow that energy to guide them from the inside-out. If one of them falls, as in becoming automatic or not hearing the music, they pause, adjust, and decide whether to continue the dance.

## PEP AND THE PLANE OF POSSIBILITY

The creative is the place where no one else has ever been.
—Alan Alda, actor[12]

I hope you now appreciate that great sex is a matter of a mind-set, not a skill set. Erotic attunement is a call-and-response between two people who are willing to meet each other with no predetermined sense of what should happen in this *particular* sexual encounter. Only when we learn to cultivate an open and curious state of mind are we able to discover "other things."

While at stage 2 we may have memorized each other's erogenous zones, at stage 3 we now view the entire body as a clean slate. We let go of our expectations of each other's turn-ons and turn-offs and meet fresh every time. It is here that stage 3 couples source a more mature and wakeful quality of enchantment than their greener stage 1 selves.

This ongoing discovery process requires being in the moment with where eros is taking us. That is why we have emphasized mindfulness practice so much. By learning to be present, curious, and empty of expectations, we enter a novelty state. In reality, though, sex for many couples has become a dance between the possible and the probable, which leads us to repeat performances of familiar moves and routines. However, the opportunities for experiencing our pure erotic potential as a couple lie in going toward what is possible and *unknown*.

In the dance between the probable and the possible, I find Dan Siegel's model of the "plane of possibility," which draws from quantum physics, to be helpful[13] (see figure 6.2, "Plane of Possibility Map"). According to Siegel, the highest point of probability is a peak of 100 percent probability of a certain action and a zero chance of the possibility of something else happening. It is when an act of remembering becomes an actual memory, or an impulse to move becomes an action. The plane goes from unformed, to forming, to fully formed, such as when a response becomes a conditioned impulse.

In contrast, a zero chance of probability (or repetition) is 100 percent possibility, or what he calls "pure awareness" to the moment. We could liken this state of pure awareness to what I call an "anything is possible" state of mind. Such a state supports the unlimited creativity of our pure erotic potential. Conversely, when habits drive our erotic behavior (100 percent probability), we will repeat the same things over and over, incurring little excitement, creativity, or novelty in bed.

While I hadn't heard of the plane of possibility when I coined the term *pure erotic potential*, it is a similar idea. We access our PEP by releasing our filters as much as we can, and we strive for a 100 percent possibility concerning erotic expression.

Some readers of a scientific bent may relate to the notion of probability more quickly than a novelty state, or pure erotic potential. The idea here is that if we are bringing awareness to the moment, without filters, then anything *is* possible when we dance with eros. Conversely, when we filter our experience with limiting mind-sets, trances, expectations, and beliefs, we find ourselves going toward our default settings automatically.

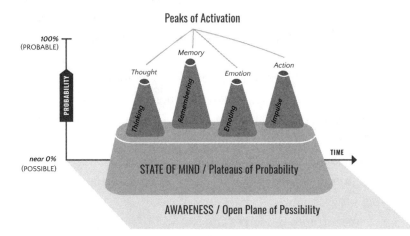

**FIGURE 6.2 PLANE OF POSSIBILITY MAP**

This map shows us how we move from an "anything is possible" state of mind (100 percent possibility on the plane of awareness) to a peak activation (100 percent probability). By working with our state of mind to remove our filters, we can follow erotic impulses born at the moment rather than relying on PEP-limiting habits and routines.

On the map of the plane of possibility (figure 6.2) Siegel illustrates these "filters" as plateaus, which are the raised platforms you can see that represent energy moving upward toward probability. Perhaps now you see why mindful sex requires being wakeful and how it can also wake us up. We have to be present and embodied to feel eros and let it lead us somewhere new. To *transform* ourselves through sex, we have to wake up to something vast, untamed, and authentic. Mindfulness practice has the potential to lay the ground for us to locate ourselves in such an unconditioned place of possibility.[14]

## THE BOTH/AND OF THE EROTIC DANCE

The good news is that we can develop our capacity for attunement through mindfulness training. Connecting to our felt sense while sensing our partner is part of the both/and approach of Passion and Presence. Thus far, we have applied that idea to the pleasure-and-pain package of sex; now, with erotic attunement, we use the concept a bit differently. How can we *both* feel ourselves—meaning our embodied presence *and* sense of direction—*and* also be in exchange with our partner?

Research shows that regular mindfulness meditation thickens the part of the brain that enables you to decipher each other's nonverbal cues.[15] This region is called the insula, and we explored it in chapters 2 and 4. The insula, along with other parts of the brain's resonance circuitry, helps us tune into our felt sense, and, in turn, feel into our partner's intentions and feelings. In this way, erotic attunement is an inside-out process.

First, we tune into ourselves and connect to our eros energy, the energy moving inside of ourselves. We sense what we are feeling and desiring in this moment and allow our bodies to move accordingly. Then we connect to our partner; we tune into what they seem to be communicating through their body. As we track them, we notice what appears inside of us in response to our partner's moves. After several back-and-forths, we can sense what is emerging between us. *We are in our pure erotic potential when we are simply in the flow of the ever-changing now rather than navigating the situation with our mind.*

With this inside-out approach, we connect to the experience that is *wanting to happen* rather than striving to make something happen. The key to erotic attunement is to feel how your eros energy wants to play through you right now, knowing this may change throughout the dance or at different stages of life. As John Welwood reminds us, a "hearty enjoyment of sex" is like the enduring pleasure of music; it happens when we immerse ourselves in the "stream of its energy, letting go, and seeing where it takes us."[16]

Speaking of music: It's a little-known fact that orchestral musicians frequently succumb to boredom because they play the same repertoire for every performance. Looking at music and mindfulness, Ellen Langer conducted an interesting study.[17] I claim the findings transfer to sex. Langer divided a sample of orchestral musicians into two groups. She asked one group to remember the best performance they ever gave of a particular composition. Then, she asked them to try to play that piece again, the same way as before. Langer told the other group to play the same composition, but to modify it in a way that only they would know. Then she recorded both performances. What were her findings? First, the musicians who improvised a tiny bit had a much better time playing the piece. They were present and responding to what felt right at the moment.

Moreover, listeners of both recordings rated the improvised piece much higher than the standard version. What does making music have to do with making love? There's evidence that improvisation enlivens all creative activities, why not sex?

## THE THREE FRIENDS: UNCERTAINTY, EMERGENCE, AND NOVELTY

> Creativity can solve almost any problem. The creative act, the defeat of habit by originality, overcomes everything.
> —George Lois[18]

If you are stuck in routine sex, trying to manipulate sex will not get you out of your rut. Nor will becoming a master of cunnilingus or fellatio or introducing a spicy role-play. A mindful approach to sex is about sensing, feeling, and responding to the elemental wild spirit of eros in a free-flowing dance. On the naked path, sex is a creative collaboration, an interplay of eros energy filtered through our shifting states and moods.

Letting eros lead replaces safety with risk and routine with uncertainty. While Henri Frédéric Amiel says, "Uncertainty is the refuge of hope,"[19] putting our hope into action is particularly vulnerable in the sexual arena. Even if we feel asphyxiated by our certain routines, we may not want to chance going freestyle. It is natural to feel anxious when we take a new turn; however, "Creativity, authenticity, uncertainty, anxiety—these cannot be separated. To live a creative existence means to live with uncertainty," claims psychotherapist and writer Kerry Gordon.[20]

Owen and Seth are bored with their sex life because their once highly arousing scenario has become a tired "get off" routine. While it appears to be edgy, the fantasy they enact is automatic, mindless, and methodical. It has become a safe place in which to hide for this very reason. Moreover, the tracks they've laid by traveling the same course so often makes the pull to go there again and again very strong.

How do we engender possibility rather than probability in our sexual encounters? I tell the couple that the rule of thumb for keeping sex fresh is to let each encounter be a "maiden voyage." When there is no template for our lovemaking, we can key off of the eros energy within and between us right now. If we try to fix eros energy to one form, we will lose touch with the capacity of sex "to renew us and illuminate the heights and depths of human experience."[21] Embracing uncertainty is how we recover the mystery that eludes us when we engage in routine-driven sex—no matter how spicy our routine is or once was.

With the aspiration to keep their dance fresh, Owen and Seth set off to find their eros energy. They begin their next erotic encounter by putting on music and let their bodies move from the inside-out, not how they dance at a club. Then, they meditate across from one another, waiting for an impulse born solely of the moment before acting. It felt awkward, they confess. However, for a full twenty minutes, they went freestyle—making eye contact and following fresh impulses to connect lovingly, roughly, playfully and creatively. Eventually, they went back to a version of their routine. Nevertheless, the old scenario felt fresh and fun because they were connected, awake, and open to letting eros lead.

As we have seen being present erotically with our scripted singular part, rather than with our whole multidimensional selves, is a way to avoid, numb, or hide deeper issues from ourselves and each other. When we bring our many selves to the exchange, we sometimes make up new movements on the spot as different parts dance in novel ways. Engaging in an unscripted exchange took Owen and Seth's relationship to another level of nakedness.

When each person's actions depend on the ones before it in a natural flow of moving energy, Erotic Attunement opens the door for Erotic Emergence. By going into the dark, with no known endpoint, we discover "other things."[22] With practice, Owen and Seth eventually gained a fair amount of comfort with Erotic Attunement. They tell me that two things have given new life to their increasingly rewarding and creative sex life. The first is having whole-person multimodal sex, where different parts play across the pyramid most every time. The second is letting eros lead.

## THE EROS CYCLE

While it's beautiful to say, "Let go of goals, and attune to eros," I'm often asked, "But, what do we actually *do* instead? How do we dance with eros in a free-flowing way?" For many people, it may even seem unimaginable to move from routine to improvisation. However, even in the arts, we have to learn to improvise; for most of us, it does not come naturally no matter the application. For this reason, I came up with a simple four-letter acronym to help you put the concept of erotic attunement into practice. I call it the EROS cycle (see figure 6.3, "EROS Cycle"). Here are the steps:

E—Embody and attune
R—Relax goals and relate
O—Open to impulses
S—Savor pleasure

And remember, stop and start over if you are becoming automatic.

## Sourcing Our Pure Erotic Potential at the Center of EROS

Before going through the four phases of EROS, I recommend that you begin by imagining the center of the cycle as the vast ocean of your PEP. The center is spacious and uncertain. It is where we empty ourselves of goals and expectations, as well as inner and outer models of what sex "should" be. Creativity starts with nothingness because in the dark is where we discover "other things." If we are filled up with our ideas about sex or preoccupied with goals and models, we can't experience anything new. For this reason, you might also imagine your PEP as "the dark."

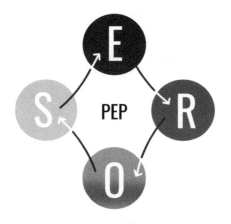

**E:** Embody & Attune
**R:** Relax Goals & Relate
**O:** Open to Impulses
**S:** Savor Pleasure

FIGURE 6.3 EROS CYCLE

The EROS cycle helps us practice the skill of erotic attunement. By mindfully moving through the four phases of the cycle, we learn to key off of our eros energy as a couple and engage in an unscripted call-and-response.

In truth, being empty and wide open can be terrifying. The "anything is possible" state is not far from the unnerving "anything can happen to me" state, which may not have such positive connotations. Understandably, we may want to return to a familiar landscape, one in which we seem to have control, can outwit pain, and avoid exposing ourselves to potentially hurtful encounters. Thus again, we find ourselves poised between possibility and probability. We long for uncertainty, but only if it is the "right" kind. "Shrinking by thinking" is one way to leave the vulnerable open space of pure potential.

While "filling up" with ideas about sex may give us a sense of protection, albeit a false one, it also comes at a high cost to our PEP. For this reason, we begin to dance by clearing the cache of our erotic history, becoming curious, and meeting fresh. This is the starting point of the EROS cycle and where we return to throughout the dance if we are becoming automatic or going toward a plateau.

## Moving Mindfully through the EROS Cycle

### E: EMBODY AND ATTUNE

After anchoring ourselves in the mind-set of our PEP, we cultivate an embodied presence to connect to our eros energy (embody and attune). I recommend that you sit opposite each other, or even lie down next to each other and practice a few minutes of mindfulness meditation together. Meditation serves as a bridge from doing to being. Then, start to scan your body from the inside out, be aware of any places of tension or unease, and let the out-breath bring relaxation and ease to the body.

## R: RELAX GOALS AND RELATE

Look at where your mind is going, consciously let go of goals, erase your templates, and anchor into the pure possibility of your PEP. You might want to create a symbol for yourself to help you do this, such as the plane of possibility map or an open sky, "the dark," or even imagining the center of the EROS cycle. Once you establish an "anything is possible" state of mind, open up to your partner by looking at them. Let your hands meet or sense each other energetically.

## O: OPEN TO IMPULSES

As you look at each other or lightly touch, individually, track your energy to locate your power source, no matter how faint. Be curious. Feel as a vessel of eros energy. Where does it live in you right now? Let yourself sense that there are endless pathways. Forget about looking good, and try not to fall back on patterned moves.

Find some way to express the energy of eros as it is there right now by opening to your impulses. (Maybe start with a small movement, a light stroke; let one movement lead to another without forcing or preempting the direction.) Join to each other with your back-and-forth moves. Allow sounds to accompany your movements if you like. Continue to feel yourself and your partner. Let eros guide you as you open to the erotic thread unfolding between you.

## S: SAVOR PLEASURE

Throughout the experience, savor pleasure in big and small ways—meaning, bring awareness to your senses and enjoy the good body feelings that you experience through moving, touching, sounding, and feeling your connection.

If you notice that you are losing connection to yourself, or falling into your routine, stop and start over. If you feel awkward, nervous, or exposed, you are doing it right.

Most importantly, use the EROS process only as a suggestion. Be playful with it and stay light on your feet. It is not meant to be a ritual to follow every time, just a way to help you get started. It can take time to break out of tried-and-true methods. At the same time, as mindful sex intends to be free rather than dogmatic, if we sometimes follow our usual course, so be it.

## The EROS Cycle: A Closer Look

Let's now look at each of the four steps of EROS more closely. Each of us might find one or more of the steps difficult or challenging. This closer look is a chance for you to sense into which of the aspects you are comfortable with now and which will require more time. I will give you suggestions for how you might work with any challenges you discover as you try this out.

Remember that erotic attunement takes practice. Even musicians learn scales and chords before they can improvise. Dancers stretch to get their bodies limber before they can flow together. Be patient with yourself and let curiosity guide you. When habits take over, let the curious mind of the "observer" study what is going on inside of you.

### E: EMBODY AND ATTUNE

After entering the center, the first phase of EROS is to cultivate an embodied presence. In the sexual arena, we are using our connection to our felt self as a compass and a guide. While we might wish that we could think our way to this energy, our ideas about sex, in fact, only get in the way. Thoughts drown out signals from the body. Instead, we need to become more sensitive to our wild elemental energy.

Unfortunately, when we are in our doing mode, we tend to disregard our bodies. We may delay sleep and urination, numb ourselves to physical pain, and stimulate ourselves with drugs to keep going. Moreover, many of us live in our heads much of the time. We may view our body as merely a transport device for our gray matter. According to the consultant and coach Julie Daley, "Awareness from the shoulders up is like living powered by a 15-watt light bulb. It makes life dim and makes it hard to experience the fullness of the world we live in."[23]

In contrast, an embodied presence is what enables you to be in contact with yourself and your partner. To become sensitive to our eros energy, we have first to notice how we deaden our bodies, effectively numbing ourselves to our power source. Is it by overeating or being sedentary, which can leave you feeling dull and sluggish? Do you live from the neck up, mostly in your head? If so, make it a practice to stop and check in with yourself throughout the day. Ask your body what it needs.

So, how can we wake up the body? You might try shaking or tapping every part of your body. You can also stretch mindfully by letting your body move you rather than trying to reproduce a yoga posture. Dancing is also a great way to come home to your body and, as we saw with Carla and Miguel, a fantastic way to wake up your many parts as well. Another option (of many) is to circle your hips and tilt your pelvis back and forth several times. Whatever you do, feel into the areas you are moving to connect to your felt sense.[24]

If you have trouble being present and embodied during sex, pause to feel yourself as often as you remember. Make eye contact with your partner whenever you can. Use mindfulness to direct attention to your physical sensations, particularly if you are getting swept into thinking. Consider sharing what you are noticing inside yourself with your partner. If your numbness is due to trauma, go back to the six ways to uncouple now from then (chapter 4).

Activities such as yoga, body-centered psychotherapy, and mindful body-scan exercises can help you learn how to check back in with your body, rather than checking out.

On the naked path, being embodied enables you to:

1. Detect and follow your eros energy;
2. Recognize somatic indicators of yes and no;
3. Observe and express your erotic impulses; and
4. Identify when and how to adjust to feel more comfortable and engaged.

## R: RELAX GOALS AND RELATE

Trust the body knows what the body wants, and allow the body
and mind to go where it feels natural.
—Dr. Martha Lee, clinical sexologist[25]

When we dance with eros, we let the reins go and trust what is emerging. If we notice we are grasping, we soften and let eros lead. Letting go involves dropping our need to perform, or to have a particular outcome; we are merely meeting what's here with a welcoming and curious presence. However, as we have seen, we need training in mindfulness to develop this quality of attention.

As mentioned, some of us lead with too firm a hand. Instead of opening up to the music, we focus only on getting our steps right. We may have trouble being spontaneous or not knowing what to do. We may find that we are straining to achieve a particular goal (such as reaching orgasm or having "great sex") and feeling anxious and pressured during sex. Moreover, as we saw with the plane of possibility map, a goal is a plateau: it ensures we will go toward probability.

If you tend to be goal oriented, let yourself empty out and assume an "anything is possible" state of mind before having sex. Start with a few minutes of mindfulness and set an intention to embrace uncertainty. Find a way to imaginatively put away your map so you can follow your curiosity. Start to engage physically with your partner from a place of interest, pausing when you don't know where to go.

When we are preoccupied with our thoughts about performance or trying to get somewhere, we disconnect from our partner. We forget this is a two-person dance and a cocreation rather than something we are solely responsible for engineering. Whenever you are observing and critiquing yourself, come into connection with your partner. Relate by making eye contact, checking in, and letting yourself feel the energy between you. You might also imagine your relationship with eros, which is moving through you and guiding your movements.

Signal your partner when you become swept up in doing, then pause, exhale, and wait for an impulse born of the moment. Don't press on—

discover something new that arises from inside. Visualize the center every time you pause. If you are thinking you should be harder, wetter, more aroused—more anything—remember that wherever you are is where you want to be. There is no end point, just this now moment.

On the naked path relaxing involves:

Relinquishing goals and reference points
Allowing rather than directing
Pausing when you're not sure where to go
Adapting to changes in your eros energies

## O: OPEN TO IMPULSES

As we feel ourselves and our eros energy and connect to our partner, we can observe impulses to move into connection. We might be moved to kiss, touch, stroke, hold each other, or make eye contact. Perhaps we want to receive some touch. For some of us, initiating is incredibly vulnerable, which, according to Brené Brown, involves uncertainty, risk, and emotional exposure.[26] It is for this reason that implementing a "no mistakes" protocol is so essential (see chapter 5).

This phase of the EROS cycle is also about responding, which can be equally vulnerable to many people. How do you meet your partner's overtures for sex? How do you "join with" their moves as in improvisation? Do you support the flowering of your partner's impulses or do you nip them in the bud by sticking to the usual script or dropping the ball? Are you so focused on your own needs that you forget this is a two-person dance? If so, slow down and pause when your partner expresses an impulse to let eros guide your next move. See if you can align your movement with theirs and engage in a little call-and-response.

Luli, a first-generation American raised by dominating parents, found this phase of the cycle to be especially challenging. Often shamed as a child for the tiniest of mistakes, she became a compliant, courteous, and sad little girl who grew up to be a sexually contained adult. Although Luli is very attuned to her body and her partner, she feels unable to express herself or take leadership, sexually. You may remember that Jerome also had difficulty expressing himself because of his hidden factors (chapter 4). He discovered that his passivity was a strategy formed in childhood to keep other people safe.

Many of us inhibit our impulses out of fear that we will make a mistake and get in trouble for it. We may not want to risk feeling incompetent or rejected. We may, like Luli, feel disempowered to shape things to our liking and inhibit sexual impulses to avoid judgment, shame, or ridicule.

If you hold back during sex, let yourself sense what your impulse might be if there were no unpleasant consequences for you. Explore what it would take for you to feel free to initiate and respond. See if you can establish some of those conditions in advance with your partner. Then, in small increments, starting with five minutes, follow the flow of energy moving through you. Become aware of the many choice points for expression and vocalize your impulses even if you choose not to act on them. Mindfully study anything that is stopping you from going toward pleasure or following your curiosity.

Through implementing such a process, Luli realized that she had trained herself to defer to others to avoid criticism. After a few of these exploratory, "fail-proof" sessions, Luli felt confident enough to engage in a more free-flowing exchange.

On the naked path, being open to impulses might include:

Initiating sex on a regular basis
Expressing impulses that emerge moment to moment
Responding to our partner's moves
Requesting things that we might like to try or receive from our
    partner

## S: SAVOR PLEASURE

Like soaking in a hot tub, pleasure rests on our ability to savor. To experience pleasure throughout the dance, we have to attune to our sensations and emotions. Pleasure typically consists of having good body feelings, but can also be a feeling of love and appreciation as we give and receive. We don't have to limit our offering to our hands. Remember, we are following our curiosity, exploring, allowing, opening to new directions.

We can help our partner "join" with us by signaling our pleasure. We can show appreciation by moaning, using words, or giving a signal like a thumbs-up when something feels right. We can also guide our partner's hand somewhere else or put our hand on theirs to show them how we want to be touched.

In my practice, I work with many people with blocks to pleasure and sexual satisfaction. For this reason, I'm going to spend a bit more time on this one. Most often, people either express disappointment around sex or feel ambivalent about their needs. Bella, a thirty-three-year-old athletically built woman, is an excellent example of someone who has trouble receiving. At stage 1 of her relationship with Ezra, Bella was able to focus on her sexual pleasure. However, now at stage 2, she feels awkward and exposed when Ezra pleasures her orally.

Most of the time, she either pushes him away or becomes the giver. She also finds it harder to orgasm this way. Like many women, Bella was raised to be "other-directed." The eldest of four sisters, Bella was used to being in the caretaking role. Her father died of a rare heart condition when she was eight years old, leaving Bella's mother in charge of everything. Bella could see how pressured her mother was by this, and did whatever she could to be helpful.

During a mindfulness homework exercise at our retreat, Bella observed her experience while receiving oral sex from Ezra. She noticed that her body was rigid and that she was worrying that Ezra was working too hard to arouse her. Later, Bella explored these feelings using mindful self-study. She imagined receiving oral sex and explored the tension this created in her body. She also noticed feelings of guilt. Bella stayed with the guilty feeling and traced it back in time. As she did this, memories slowly came into view of her mother crying at the dining table. Bella remembers feeling anxious that her mother would also die if things became too much for her. This fear strengthened the young Bella's not-fully conscious resolve to ignore her own needs.

Bella and Ezra did a few sessions of mindful coinvestigation in which Ezra gave Bella oral sex for three to five minutes, with no goal of bringing her to orgasm. Bella chose to stay with her discomfort rather than deflecting attention away from herself. She agreed to pause and let Ezra know when she was getting tense, and to check in with him every time. This exercise in teaming up helped Bella see that Ezra felt nourished by pleasuring her rather than burdened. Over time, Bella was able to receive pleasure from oral sex again.

Perhaps like Judith, it seems like nothing your partner does is ever good enough. In confidence, Judith tells me that Frank "just doesn't know what he is doing," even though she has instructed him many times. This admission came after she complained that Frank never wants sex, although she failed to see the connection between her criticism and his avoidance. I recommended the following mindful coinvestigation activity:

I told Judith to take a moment to feel into herself and ask her body what kind of touch it would like to receive. Then, I encouraged her to let Frank provide this touch for no more than two minutes. "Coach him, so he gets the touch just right," I said, "Then, mindfully study anything that stops you from enjoying the experience." A mindful approach is not about overcoming our barriers; it is about replacing automaticity with awareness.

Judith came into her next session, humbled by her discoveries. "It's me; not Frank," she blurted. "I told Frank exactly what to do, and he did it just right, but somehow I couldn't relax into it. I kept scanning for problems. First, the room was too cold; then, I wanted Frank to be more connected. Eventually, I realized that no matter what we did to make things better, I still couldn't enjoy it." I told Judith that sex sometimes puts a spotlight on things that are shaping us outside of awareness. It is natural to want to blame our partner, but often an internal prohibition is preventing us from receiving the very thing that we want.

Over the next few weeks, Judith realized that underneath her critical protector was a part that didn't feel deserving of pleasure. As we did more inner work to uncover the experiences that had informed this implicit "knowledge," Judith did another mindfulness activity with Frank. She agreed to put her attention toward what is right and satisfying, no matter how small, and to let it nourish her. A few months later, Judith sheepishly told me that Frank was a pretty good lover after all. Your lover might be too if you can let yourself take in the nourishment.

On the naked path, we savor pleasure by:

Opening to our bodily sensations
Giving and receiving pleasure as a mutual exchange
Feeling gratitude for the good feelings we are experiencing
Letting things be "good enough" rather than perfect

## THE NAKED PAUSE

At stage 3, we continue to use the erotic portal for growth, even when we use EROS. At any time, we can shift from "having sex," to stopping to explore anything that seems to interfere with our ability to attune to ourselves or our partner. We use our observer to detect instances where we seem to be disengaging from our felt sense, going into performance mode, inhibiting impulses, and blocking pleasure. If you want to shift rather than strengthen those habits, take a "naked pause." Here there are two options: stop and start over, or stop and study.

These tendencies may relate to any of the PEP barriers we have looked at so far: automaticity, trance states, fear of vulnerability, the hidden factors, or shame. Moreover, repetition, leading to habits of body and mind, is perhaps the most significant barrier to our PEP. Though we may long for new vistas, we will forever take the same roads if we are asleep at the wheel. It is for this reason that being wakeful is necessary to restore the creativity that gets lost in our long-term relationship. Therefore, we want to pause whenever we notice we are:

1. Going on automatic
2. Becoming uncomfortable or losing aliveness
3. Unsure of where to go next
4. Being goal oriented
5. Straining—to get into sex, climax, or please our partner
6. Distracted or preoccupied
7. Judging our self, our partner, or the experience
8. Triggered in any way
9. Following a script or defaulting to a numbing routine

Each time you pause, either study and share, or adjust and anchor back into your PEP at the center of the cycle—that is, the place of openness, uncertainty, and 100 percent possibility. Then, wait for an eros-led impulse.

## IT'S OKAY TO STEP ON EACH OTHER'S TOES

A person who never made a mistake never tried anything new.
—Albert Einstein[27]

When we let eros lead, we maintain a curious, open presence. We become a witness, rather than a director. From this embodied state, "the dancer dances." As mentioned earlier, many of us have trouble relaxing. We worry that we will make a mistake and mess up the dance. Marty Klein, the author of *Sexual Intelligence*, says: "One of the wonderful things about sex is that we can make it a place where mistakes are not possible, and where virtually nothing can go wrong—not because we become sexually perfect, but because we radically redefine sexual 'success.'"[28]

I love this quote and encourage you to embrace the reassuring notion of "success, no matter what." In truth, though, some dances are better than others. Perhaps in this dance, we had trouble finding our stride, our rhythm was off, or we lost our balance and stepped on each other's toes. Here's how Ed Tronic, the developmental psychologist we heard about in chapter 3, describes how we dance in real life, which applies to our real-life sex:

"Unlike Fred and Ginger's dance, our dancing is hardly perfect; there are missteps, apologies, tries, retries, match-ups, and missteps again." He goes on to describe how our dancing cycles between being matched or coordinated when we are synchronous and in states of shared meanings and intentionality to mismatched or mis-coordinated when we are in dys-synchronous states. And then we can cycle back to matching intentional states via an active, jointly carried out reparatory process.[29]

So, what does this say about erotic attunement? For starters, we will misstep, not occasionally but often. We are also likely to step on each other's toes, especially when we take risks. In the movies, we see only perfect performances. In real life, we accidentally pull each other's hair, pass gas, or miss each other's cues. Instead of viewing these missteps as disastrous, we can laugh, repair, and "dance on."

## Sara and Jerry: Putting EROS into practice

Like Owen and Seth, Sara and Jerry also had a routine. Theirs was to avoid sex altogether. Openly affectionate, the love between this sixty-something couple is overflowing. They cuddle, hug, spoon, and laugh a lot. However, when Sara's libido flatlined after menopause and Jerry lost confidence in his ability to perform, eros left their bedroom.

Many couples that I work with, particularly in their fifties and sixties, stop having sex when their bodies change instead of changing or dispensing with their script. Sara decided on a yoga retreat that she wasn't ready to say goodbye to eros. Her daily walks in nature woke up a longing to explore being alive again, not just in her heart and spirit, but also in her animal body.

It was nightfall when Sara returned from the retreat, and Jerry was already sleeping, face down. She paused in the dark, taking a few moments to establish an embodied presence. For a second, Sara waivered, flashes of disappointing attempts to find their way into a satisfying erotic connection playing through her mind. Sara released them, coming back to the center—she got mindful and embraced the uncertainty of the dark.

Sara looked at Jerry and waited for an impulse. She felt her connection to herself and also to this man who looked so innocent as he slumbered. Suddenly Sara felt guided to lie on top of him, spread eagle. She began kissing the back of Jerry's neck. He turned around, wide-eyed, and she put her finger on his lips. "I love you," she said and ran her mouth down the backside of his body. Her inner seductress came to life, and Sara found herself teasing Jerry. When he flipped over, she put his hand on her breast. To their surprise, Jerry's penis responded. After about ten minutes, their eros energy waned. Sara gave Jerry a full-body hug and snuggled against his chest. Minutes later, they were both asleep.

The next morning, Sara could still feel some eros energy rumbling inside of her. She sensed into this energy as she once again sensed her connection to Jerry, who was lying on his side, smiling. She repositioned herself so her body made a sawing motion over the ridge of his hip, and Sara began to hum. She was not humming a particular tune, just a made-up melody. Jerry started moaning, in resonance, and then his animal woke up. He growled and scratched the inside of Sara's arms. His teeth made tiny bites along the inside of her wrist and under her breasts. Then he nipped at her neck. Both found these unscripted moves to be very exciting.

The energy turned playful then, and both started to wrestle. The couple giggled and good-naturedly jostled until Jerry collapsed onto Sara's belly. He rested his hand on her mons pubis, and she began rocking her hips, pressing her pelvis into his still hand. Jerry brushed his hair against Sara's stomach by moving his head in a sweeping motion and shot out little puffs of air over her belly, something he had never done before.

Sara tells me she began to shiver, laugh, and cry all at once. Then Jerry started to stimulate her orally. Midway through, she signaled for him to pause. Sara recognized that this was a common arousal pathway and definite plateau. Customarily, she would call up an arousing fantasy to bring herself to orgasm; however, Sara wanted to stay in the open space of her pure erotic potential.

For a moment, Sara felt lost and started to worry, then she felt into herself and let her body guide her next move. Sara tells me she was in an altered state and can't remember everything. It was like her thinking brain shut down, and her body was moving her toward pleasure in ways that even her younger self had never known. "I was looking out at the sky through our Palladian window. There was the slightest frost on the trees, but the sky was very blue. Something inside of me felt trustworthy, like I really could take the oars out of the water."

As Sara is speaking, I am struck by how vibrant she looks, whereas only a few weeks earlier, she appeared to be "grayed out." She continues, "It wasn't about having an orgasm or looking sexy; it was like you said, 'letting the energy move me in new ways.' I lay on top of Jerry and let my entire body feel the warmth from his skin. I breathed him in and just let myself rock gently on top of him. Jerry started to sway, too, and it was so soothing and innocent."

Without overthinking it, Sara reached for the Pulse, which is a sex toy for men (affectionately known as the "guybrator").[30] Jerry didn't resist, although the toy had lain in the drawer unused for a couple of months. It turned out to be incredibly arousing, and Jerry climaxed within minutes. This post-orgasm phase would typically be another plateau, a time to rearrange themselves into their habitual roles. Sara was curious to see what would happen if she continued to listen inside and wait for the next impulse.

When it came, Sara asked Jerry to kiss her. The kissing grew in intensity, and Sara started rubbing herself against Jerry's front body in a rocking motion. Jerry supported the rocking with his hands, and his breath quickened as he felt Sara's mounting excitement. As the energy peaked, Jerry glided his hands from Sara's back to her buttocks and then slipped a finger inside of her anus. She let out a little gasp and was surprised when she had an orgasm from merely rocking her pelvis against Jerry's right thigh.

Jerry chimes in now to tell me how much he loved that Sara took charge and that his focus was not just on his "equipment." Usually, he would be inside a small "worry bubble," unable to feel much of himself or tune into his wife. Before that lovemaking adventure, he had been too embarrassed to use the toy and still wasn't sure how often he wanted to use it in the future. However, in the heat of the moment, his self-consciousness fell away, and it was fun to enjoy the vibrating sensations.

Before leaving, Sara says, "It was thrilling to liberate myself from the old script. I now understand what you mean by an 'anything is possible' state of mind. The way we were together was so much more enlivening than trying to work to get aroused and have an orgasm." Jerry is blushing as he listens to Sara's graphic report, though his head is nodding and he can't help but smile.

Uncertainty can usher us into sexual experiences of a new and different order. Such encounters are wholly unique, unrepeatable, and radically novel. The trick is to stay open and exploratory, rather than to fall back into routines that stifle our pure erotic potential. When we catch the impulse to repeat our usual moves and instead take a new turn, sex, like life itself, becomes more interesting—even sizzling—on occasion.

## MINDFUL ACTIVITIES AND NAKED REFLECTIONS

### Moving Mindfully through the EROS Cycle

Take some time to reflect on the EROS cycle. How might you help yourselves to anchor into the center of your PEP when you make love? Which of the other four phases are natural, and which ones do you know or imagine are challenging for you?

Plan a time when you will try out the EROS cycle. See if your self-assessment about each phase was correct. What might you do to bring more awareness to the areas that are challenging to you? Consider trying out the exploratory exercises listed in the chapter.

### Naked Reflections

In what ways are you caught in a performance mind-set? What is your "internal model"—your habitual way of making love—that you keep steering toward automatically? What fears and concerns do you have about erotic attunement? How can you support each other in letting eros lead, in sensing and surrendering to this energetic power? How can you give yourselves permission to step on each other's toes?

# 7.

# EROTIC SUSTENANCE

## Tending Our Magic through the Seasons

> When two people meet and fall in love, there's a sudden rush of magic. Magic is just naturally present then. We tend to feed on that gratuitous magic without striving to make any more.
>
> —TOM ROBBINS[1]

What does the naked path look like as we head into our golden years? Can we have a vital erotic life as we age and become ever more familiar with one another? Can working with our consciousness keep sex fresh over many decades, or do we have to do something else to keep eros alive?

The word *sustenance* comes from the word *sustain*, which means "to continue." While modern pharmacology can restore flagging hormones to near pubescent levels, sex is more than a physical act. As I indicated in chapter 6, sex is a dance with mystery, an intimate expression of our life force as it plays through us right here, right now. To sustain our erotic power lifelong, we must tend this energy individually and as a couple in an ongoing way.

Tending is a way to preserve eros—without putting it in a museum—so it will delight, inspire, and reward you in the years to come. For this, we must make magic in the middle and end of our journey. Preserving a long-term erotic relationship, therefore, requires relinquishing the idea that sex should always be unplanned, spontaneous, and maintenance free. Stage 3 couples engage in activities that provide "sustenance" to eros so they can bear the fruit of their endeavors and continue to receive sexual nourishment as they age.

This aim can be hard to imagine if our vision of sex requires boatloads of vigor, good looks, and a hearty libido. Because of decreasing hormone levels, as well as illness and the medications used to treat them, libido may flag in later life, if not sooner. Physical pain may make certain positions or activities impossible. We may feel less attractive and less confident in our abilities to arouse our partner or to become aroused. Thus, our sustenance plan requires a vision of eros that changes as we change and fits our current capacities and desires.

Often when it comes to sex, we find ourselves looking backward to how it once was. We either long to return there or harbor regrets for what we didn't have—such as more partners, adventures, or even satisfying experiences. Although we can't go back in time, we can step out of numbing routines—today and always. We can become mindfully and sensually embodied no matter our age or years together.

Moreover, the slow fade of sex in long-term relationships is not inevitable unless our script leads only to orgasm, and to penetration as well. Then, we may indeed find that path narrowing later in life. Also, if we believe sex is an extreme sport that requires daring stunts, we may write it out of our lives. Good sex need not be acrobatic, nor require volumes of stamina, flexibility, and grace. However, most people fix their ideas about sex, which sets them up for a sense of failure and disappointment. "Pursuing a sexual vision that's fifteen years out of date (and performing poorly at it!) isn't a dysfunction," says Marty Klein. "It's a cruel and culturally and psychologically driven mistake."[2]

As we have seen, mainstream models of sexuality fixate on performance and penetration—a reflection of our goal-driven culture and the medicalization of male sexuality.[3] Without deconstructing these models, it's hard not to feel that we have to "settle for less" if we experience declines in genital function. It might seem like the best we can hope for is to be able to cope with our chronic pain and illness and live with a sex life that feels too small. Yet by transcending the standard frame around sexuality we can potentially open as couples—whether in illness, pain, aging, fatigue, stress, or overfamiliarity—to new levels of intimacy.

A good vision inspires and also prepares us for real life. At certain times, when we are healing, for example, eros energy is more a delicate orchid than a hardy perennial. Can we dance with these changes as we dance with eros? The vision I am proposing is not just for elder sex. It involves adjusting to the various seasons of our life, the ebb and flow of eros during illness, parenting, periods of personal renewal, *and* aging. Like wintertime, some of these seasons are fallow, and eros may go into a hibernation period before reawakening in spring.

What about the transformational aspect of our vision? How do we stay awake to the ever-changing now? Can we continue to update our files about our self, our partner, and sex so that we stay awake to the possible and not default to the probable? We need an eros-sustenance plan that is grounded and embodied, and also inspires us to work with our mind rather than identifying with limiting mind-sets. Eros energy is the fuel for our conscious journey. Where can this journey take us? We will end this chapter, and thus the book, by looking at transformation in the broadest sense, beyond healing imprints and wounds—sex that changes our consciousness entirely.

## EXPANSION AND CONTRACTION: THE CONSCIOUS COUPLE'S EROTIC JOURNEY

> When you have an issue in your life, the point is not to get rid of it. The point is to grow with it.
> —A. H. Almaas[4]

Enchantment is a great feeling, but none of us can stay there. Nature has cycles, light and dark. At stage 1, our sex was hot, spontaneous, and relatively easy. Our attraction was magnetizing. We were disinhibited because we were naive. We didn't have to skirt danger; we were embold-ened to take risks. At stage 2, the incendiary powers of our attraction burned out. We wrestled with differing sexual appetites and styles, life stresses, and our hidden factors. Sex became lackluster, complicated, and triggering. When it comes down to it, at this point most of us thought there were only two available choices: to separate or go to sleep—literally and metaphorically. Hopefully now you feel confident to make the third choice: to awaken.

Sex is complicated, and it becomes even more so over time. We all face stress, illness, and aging. Moreover, demanding roles keep us in states of mobilization that are anathema to sensual arousal. Because of this, we can never continually inhabit a peak experience sexually, nor is it a matter of "willing" ourselves to stay there. Some of the challenges we face throughout life are not problems per se but are ongoing situations that we have to find ways to "live with." It is for this reason that the emphasis in this book is on developing a lifelong practice of awakened intimacy, not a one-off solution to our problems.

At stage 3, we have incorporated this perspective and no longer see life as a bed of roses as we did at stage 1. Nor do we see it as a thicket of thorns, as it seemed at stage 2. Instead, we recognize that both the flower and stem are part of the rose. Couples that transition to stage 3 have weathered storms and know they can survive more of them. They accept that impermanence, imperfection, and variability are integral features of their lives, including their sex lives.

While at stage 1 we believed ardor would inoculate us against future challenges, now we know that relationships don't (or can't) work that way. Long-term couples rarely experience an abiding sense of connection. Between periods of deep love and respect are phases of turmoil and disconnection that significantly test their resilience. This constant fluctuation between satisfaction and dissatisfaction, ease and challenge, is a feature of all living systems. It is also the evolutionary calling card for growth.

David Schnarch was the first person to apply these "facts of life" to sex. From the beginning, he has claimed that sexual problems are the engine for growth.[5] Thus, we can expect that restive periods of boredom, uncertainty, and physical discomfort will alternate with periods of calm and flow. As Michael Metz and Barry McCarthy, the authors of *Enduring Desire*, have put it, "Healthy sexuality embraces this constant

| STAGE 1 | STAGE 2 | STAGE 3 |
|---|---|---|
| • Hot and Heavy | • Lackluster | • Variable (tender, lusty, naughty, playful) |
| • Easy | • Complicated | • Cooperative |
| • Mutual Desire | • Desire Descrepancy | • Willingness |
| • Exciting, Novel | • Predictable, Routine | • State of Novelty (Meeting Fresh) |
| • Uninhibited | • Cautious, Safe | • Naked |
| • Magnetic | • Aversive, Triggering | • All-Encompassing |
| • Uncertain, Mysterious | • Familiar Arousal Pathways | • Ever-Widening Arousal Pathways |
| • Unscripted | • Scripted | • Improvised |
| • Goal-Oriented | • Goal-Oriented | • Exploratory |

FIGURE 7.1 SEX AT EACH STAGE

This table shows how we experience sex at the three stages of erotic coupling (i.e., enchantment, disenchantment, and re-enchantment.)

change, adapts to it, savors the moments of stability, and celebrates life's challenges and shifting dimensions."[6]

No one is immune to life's ripening process. Moreover, there is no endpoint at which we arrive, no peaceful, steady state. In practical terms, there will always be another pass to cross that is as steep and winding as the last one. We can defend against pain and avoid growth by closing off to life, or we can use the skills we have learned here to expand our PEP forever (refer to figure 1.1).

## A VISION OF RE-ENCHANTMENT: SEX AT STAGE 3

So, what is sex like at stage 3? As you might expect, it is variable (see figure 7.1, "Sex at Each Stage"). Because eros energy changes, our exchange may go from wild and lustful, to tender and playful. We continuously go to the center of our PEP to erase models and templates so we can enter fresh. We follow impulses that arise organically, which means our sexual encounters are unpredictable, not perfect. They can be exciting and edgy, and occasionally dull and uninspired.

At stage 3, we are not entirely immune to the deadening effect of our trance states or the remnants of our early learning. However, we orient to eros differently than at stage 1 or 2. We practice *response-agility* often. As we saw in chapter 4, we can pause, adjust, and plant hearts when we become triggered unexpectedly during sex. We are no longer afraid of what black light syndrome might reveal to us because we view the revelation of our hidden factors as an opportunity for healing and growth.

We are cooperative, which means we are considerate of each other's vulnerabilities. We check in regularly and ask for consent when we sail into unknown waters. We are committed to expanding rather than repeating old moves or playing it safe. Our dance is unscripted, and sometimes one of us is enjoying it more than the other. We take turns leading and following. If we are goal oriented, we let go and do something else. When old patterns are taking us down familiar paths, we pause and bring more presence to the connection. We switch into a novelty state whenever automaticity is robbing us of full engagement. We also cultivate the *willingness* to be sexual rather than waiting to be "in the mood."

That said, sometimes we don't have any sex at all.

## Fasting as Rest and Renewal

Shay walks into my office and throws herself onto my couch somewhat dramatically. "Life is so much better on sex!" she marvels. She's right, and we have the science to prove it. There are so many good reasons to have sex. It produces endorphins, boosts immune functioning, helps with sleep, and may lower your risk for cancer and heart attack.[7] It's like getting an oil change on your car. Afterward, the car runs better and feels better to drive. However, when Shay was exhausted from taking care of young children, her mind couldn't be further away from sex. "Truthfully, I think I'd be okay if I never had sex again," Shay insisted during the two-year dry spell she came out of recently.

Being an erotic team does not require continuous sexual engagement—everything in nature ebbs and flows. Sometimes we need to draw into ourselves to protect whatever is emerging. Returning to an individual state, rather than exchanging eros energy, can help us come home to our heart when we have strayed too far from our center.

Likewise, a physical illness may require abstinence from partner sex, or we may be put off by sex when we are breastfeeding or grieving a loss. Learning to trust that all living systems need periods of rest for renewal can quell anxiety about a "dry spell." We can explore fallow periods together and employ strategies that take care of both partners during such times.

I ask Shay how things are better now that she's having sex again. "I feel more connected to myself and in flow with life," Shay answers enthusiastically. "I'm also more open and playful with Leif, and we fight a lot less." She pauses to think for a moment, then adds, "I feel on solid ground in my relationship, allied, close, appreciative." Indeed, sexual satisfaction increases relationship satisfaction,[8] a theme we will see throughout this chapter.

So, how did Shay and Leif cope with that period of sexual inactivity? They talked about it a lot. They expressed their feelings without blaming each other. They were able to hold their pains with their hands clasped, which created a sense of being in it together. Although Shay was not interested in sex, she did sometimes pleasure Leif. Also, she was open to having her scalp massaged, even when she was touch-saturated from nursing her infant daughter. Sometimes, they held each other through the night.

"Those activities saved us," says Shay, and it's quite possibly true. In a study of hundreds of couples in five countries (Japan, Germany, Brazil, Spain, and the United States), kissing, hugging, and cuddling regularly were crucial factors in relationship satisfaction. This finding was especially true for men, which the researchers found surprising.[9]

## Body Sustenance: Tending Ourselves as Erotic Vessels

While it may not seem fun or sexy to focus on our physical health, that's where the magic starts. If eros plays through us, then the music we make depends a lot on how well we take care of ourselves. With proper fuel, adequate sleep, and exercise, our body can do remarkable things for us. If we neglect our body, it will age quicker, and more than likely, become a source of pain rather than pleasure.

These simple truths regarding physical health hold for sexual health as well. Adequate sleep, sound nutrition, and moderate exercise are the "superfoods" of our eros-sustenance plan. Many "lifestyle diseases," such as diabetes, heart disease, obesity, and high cholesterol, also have sexual side effects. As is now commonly understood, the good news is that we can often manage these conditions by changing our diet and exercising.

In terms of physical capacity, we need to "use it or lose it," regardless of illness, pain, or aging. Just as hunger signals switch off after a few days of fasting, sexual messages turn off when we fast from sex. Shay realizes now that her interest in sex *diminished* the longer she went without it. People who experience pleasurable sexual encounters, alone, and with each other, tend to want sex more. When the body wakes up, it starts speaking again. Moreover, having long gaps between sexual encounters can generate anxiety about reconnecting.

Sexual activity has other magical powers. It increases blood circulation in the genitals. Stimulating the genitals to the point of engorgement can produce stronger erections and reverse penile shrinkage after radiation or prostatectomy. It also reverses vaginal atrophy, which is the thinning, drying, and inflammation of the vaginal walls after menopause, hysterectomy, or treatment for cancer.[10]

While we may not have considered this, we can also tend our genital health. Many physical therapists specialize in strengthening or loosening the pelvic floor, which can relieve pain with penetration. Doing Kegels can lead to stronger orgasms and reduce problems with incontinence for women and men who have lax muscles in their pelvic floor.

Jade egg practices are controversial, though purported by some to be a way to keep the vagina limber, agile, and flexible. You might want to put these delicacies on your magic-making menu if they would be beneficial. Get to know your body—its needs and desires—and tend to your genital health as you tend to the rest of your body.

Another way to tend to your erotic vessel is to exercise. Sitting eight or more hours a day not only increases your risk for "lifestyle diseases" but also deadens eros.[11] It also increases anxiety, which for many of us could be beneficially decreased. Yet it is also true that each of us has an optimal zone of arousal where "anxiety" can feel like too little (say boredom or feeling too easygoing) or too much (like feelings of panic). Anxiety can also feel anywhere from tense to confident or excited.

Paying attention to your own experience of anxiety in the moment can help you determine whether exercising before sex will help or hinder your arousal. This optimal zone of functioning was first noticed in the sports arena, and varies from one athlete to another.[12] Psychotherapy uses a similar model called the window of tolerance.[13] I am using this notion in describing the "sweet spot" of safety and arousal, and closeness and desire.

Numerous studies show that women with low or average baseline levels of sympathetic nervous system (SNS) activation benefit from twenty minutes of exercise before sex.[14] Low SNS activation is associated with arousal problems and an inability to orgasm.[15] If you experience sexual side effects from antidepressants or have lower levels of estrogen due to hysterectomy or menopause, then exercise will boost your arousal.[16]

However, just like the optimal zone of performance mentioned earlier, exercising before sex can *lower* physiological sexual arousal in women with high baseline levels of SNS activity.[17] If you suffer from anxiety or have experienced childhood sexual abuse, your SNS probably runs high. Instead of exercising before sex, do something calming, such as gentle stretching, massage, deep breathing, or progressive relaxation.

You may choose to practice a form of pranayama (yogic breathing) called the 2-1 breath, where the length of the exhale is double the length of the inhale.[18] The 2-1 breath makes us feel calmer by engaging our quieting parasympathetic nervous system. Meditation also lowers our anxiety, pulse rate, and cortisol levels, which can help us downtick our nervous system before having sex. If you are not sure what is going to work best, I encourage you to experiment.

Yoga is especially good sustenance for eros because it helps you focus on how your body feels rather than how it looks. Studies show that yoga with a mindful component can help with desire, arousal, lubrication, orgasm, satisfaction, and pain, which is not the case with other forms of exercise.[19] However, all types of exercise can improve body image, which increases sexual pleasure, sexual assertiveness, and self-esteem.[20]

Poor body image does the opposite and leads to sexual avoidance.[21] It is important to note that how we see ourselves matters more than our actual size. Although a "fat-shaming" culture can have a detrimental effect on how people perceive their sexual desirability, even people of average or low weight are vulnerable to viewing themselves as sexually undesirable.[22] With so much emphasis on a small bandwidth of what "looks sexy," it can be hard to see ourselves reflected in the popular cultural images that bombard us daily.

Switching our orientation from trying to *look sexy* to *feeling sexual* is critical, especially as we age. As Klein says: "Anyone over 35, and especially those dealing with health challenges, have to empower themselves to redefine 'sexy' to include someone—yourself—in a physical state that society specifically defines as *unsexy.*"[23] Reorienting our perception in this way is key to lifelong sexual engagement.

If you worry that you've aged out of sex, or are otherwise now unworthy or unsuitable, consider this: David Schnarch, the author of *Passionate Marriage*, asserts that sex can get better as our physical capacity dims, particularly as we age. Why? Because the people who are having it grow and evolve. An older and hopefully wiser person can bring more of themselves to the experience. "People confuse genital prime with sexual prime," claims Schnarch.[24] What he means is that older people have a much higher capacity for intimacy than teenagers and young adults, which is why he insists that "cellulite and sexual potential are highly correlated."[25]

## Spiritual and Erotic Expansion in the Face of Illness and Pain

There's no denying that chronic illness and pain can bring in their wake a loss of sexual desire, as well as diminished physical functioning. Medical diseases are another one of Cupid's leaden arrows that can compromise erotic vitality by disrupting arousal and orgasm. While few, if any, chronic illnesses require a restriction of sexual activity, many people with cancer, cardiovascular disease, musculoskeletal disease, chronic respiratory disease, or HIV/AIDS stop having sex.

There are many reasons for this, including body-image concerns after surgery, as well as depression, fatigue, pain, stress, anxiety, and loss of libido. However, touch and physical intimacy are essential for everyone, including and perhaps especially those who are severely debilitated or terminally ill. As mentioned earlier, it is the bedrock of relationship satisfaction.

Although sexual side effects are painful for both partners, profound truths are often a paradox. Chronic pain and illness can weaken our body and sexual desire, and simultaneously strengthen our spiritual core by showing us that we are "not this body."

At the same time, when we let go of our models of functional sex, we can be erotic no matter how well we are functioning. That is, as our bodies ebb, eros can still flow. Living with chronic illness and pain or their aftermaths can thus become an opportunity to widen the frame of "real sex" and practice a mind-set of mindfulness. Such a mind-set worked like magic for Maurice and Angela.

Twelve months after Maurice underwent radiation treatment for prostate cancer, he struggled with erectile dysfunction that worsened over time. He could orgasm but was unable to have penetrative sex. Moreover, the medication he was taking, a type of "androgen deprivation therapy," suppresses testosterone, so he also lost his drive.[26] Disheartened and ashamed, Maurice pretty well assumed that his sex life was over.

Angela was more hopeful, although she had trouble convincing Maurice that they could gratify each other physically without an erect penis. At our couple's retreat, Maurice learned how to view the whole body as an erogenous zone. He discovered that he enjoyed intimate sensual touch on the inside of his arms and legs, that became more erotic as he "wired in" this arousal pathway. In our private session, we discussed ways to fulfill Angela's occasional desire for penetration through a strap-on, fingering, and handheld dildos.

As they expanded their sexual script and adjusted their roles, Maurice and Angela felt more intimate than ever. They learned to have naked conversations that deepened their emotional and erotic connection. Now, eight years later, they flirt, touch often, and are still expanding erotically as a couple.

## Embracing Whole-Body Sex

Sometimes cisgender, heterosexual men ask me if Passion and Presence is a female model of sex. What they usually mean is that while they think of sex as intercourse, my definition is much broader. They are correct. Any touch, movement, or exchange of energy that is pleasurable, arousing, creative, or connecting is sex in my book. When we put a wide margin around sex, it becomes inclusive to people of all abilities, body types, ages, genders, and persuasions.

Goal-oriented models that focus on penetration don't serve people with penises well. They contribute to performance anxiety and lead to avoidance, especially in cases of erectile dysfunction.[27] More importantly, they limit the amount of pleasure that people with penises can feel because they focus primarily on the genitalia. "To have truly embodied and ultimately out-of-body sex, a man has to become more attuned to his entire body, head to head and nape to toe," says Ian Kerner.[28]

Equating sex with penetrative intercourse is the most miniature view we can have of sex. It is the only kind of sex that requires birth control or an erection, says Marty Klein, and it is not an easy way for women to orgasm.[29] If "real sex" means penetration by a penis, then you will not be able to have sex if illness or age prevent you or your partner from having an erection, to say nothing of whether one of the partners has a penis. It seems timely to unseat penile penetration from the sexual throne. I want you to be sexual as long as you want to be, in whatever form that takes.

Michael Metz and Barry McCarthy are also in this camp. They developed a model of sexuality for midlife men experiencing erectile dysfunction called good enough sex (GES).[30] While the name sounds like mediocre sex is the best you can hope for, GES really is about realistically great sex. The model encourages men to widen the frame from penis/vagina sex to include a wide range of arousal pathways, and to privilege pleasure over performance.

I like to think of this widening more as embracing whole-body sex. I encourage you to expand your repertoire from penis/vagina or penis/

anus sex and to view your entire body as an erogenous zone. Be open to including hugging, touching, massage, self-stimulation, the use of sex toys and vibrators, mutual masturbation, oral sex, as well as playing with fantasies, and to considering these activities to be "real sex."

## Relationships Need Tending Too: Conscious Covenants for Your Erotic Team

How did Angela and Maurice's sex life improve over time? Besides widening the frame of what "real sex" is they also worked diligently to tend their relationship. A cooperative alliance is our vehicle for navigating the naked path. Appreciation for each partner's willingness to be on this journey to be naked is how we remain a cooperative and engaged erotic team.

We cannot assume that intimacy is self-sustaining, either. A cooperative alliance involves having a shared direction and path to become wakeful, as we work with challenges and nurture our relationship. Such an alliance requires time and care. For starters, we might create a covenant that includes our aspirations for tending eros together. Below is a covenant that Maurice and Angela swear by. They claim that adhering to their covenant has improved their sex life and strengthened their relationship core. Perhaps a covenant will do the same for you.

As you can see, their covenant incorporates the key components of the naked path. If you fashion such an agreement, pick and choose what suits you and add other items that matter to you that are not on this list. Periodically review your covenant to see if it needs revision and explore how well you are meeting your aspirations.

### SOME KEY INGREDIENTS OF A RELATIONAL COVENANT

We establish an eros-sustenance plan that includes taking care of ourselves mentally, physically, and sexually

We clear whatever is coming between us, so we are open to sex

We get naked with each other, both emotionally and erotically

We talk openly about our desires and fears with curiosity and compassion

When problems arise, we address them with clasped hands

We avoid blaming one another when things don't go right

We commit to expanding the "us" zone of our Venn diagram

We repair ruptures and restore trust when needed

We create a container in which it is safe to take risks sexually and emotionally

We view challenges as catalysts for growth

We use our erotic relationship to heal and transform

We revise our implicit and explicit agreements as necessary

We schedule erotic dates

We take responsibility for our arousal rather than expecting our partner to do all the work

We explore triggers with mindful coinvestigation

We both initiate sex and cultivate a willingness to be erotic together

We practice seeing fresh, touching fresh, and meeting fresh

We actively develop a state of "connected longing" (see below)

Individually:

We do additional work, as needed, to work with erotic wounds from our past

We each have a regular mindfulness practice to widen our tolerance for uncertainty, hear each other without becoming reactive, and cultivate presence and curiosity

We explore our triggers and aversions through mindful self-study

We get to know our protector and protected parts

We get radically naked by showing what we most want to hide

## Making Time for Fun, Sex, and Romance

Sometimes it seems that we provide the best of ourselves to our children, colleagues, and friends, dropping "the mask" for our beloved. While it is comforting to be "real," by not putting on airs with each other, exchanging patience, kindness, and generosity can be the magic that opens us to sex.

At the same time, we may falsely assume we have to improve our relationship before we can be sexual with one another. If you view sex as the icing on a cake that has already fallen, it may hearten you to know that you don't have to strengthen each layer before enjoying the cream. Many couples find that once they nurture their erotic relationship that—like magic—they get along better. Indeed, studies indicate that sexual satisfaction increases relationship satisfaction, though the reverse is not always the case.[31]

Unfortunately, it's hard to revitalize eros when we're entrenched in our regular patterns. We have to pause long enough to reverse the negative spiral of being too stressed to nurture our erotic connection and too tired to be nurtured by it. I recommend getting away once or twice a year, if possible, to do a relationship "reset." During this time, focus only on each other. Avoid doing email on your retreat and practice seeing and meeting fresh continuously. Set aside time to be erotic every day.

You can also do the activities at the end of this chapter on your retreats. In between these retreats, try to schedule three other kinds of dates: fun and romance dates, erotic dates, and tending dates. Let's look at each of these in turn.

## FUN AND ROMANCE DATES (WEEKLY OR BIWEEKLY)

These dates take place outside of the house. The intent is to de-role from our eros-diminishing parts and focus on each other in the ways you did at stage 1. Back then, you listened attentively, and with curiosity. You shared your hopes and dreams, how good you feel in the other's company, what fun things you might do together in the weeks to come. You made eye contact, touched, and smiled often. You didn't talk about problems at work, money woes, difficulties with your children, or in-laws.

All of that "maintenance" stuff enrolls you as domestic managers to each other rather than lovers. It is the de-eroticizing aspect of what Cheryl Fraser, the author of *Buddha's Bedroom*, calls "Marriage Inc."[32] Instead of having a business meeting, let yourself go back to the early days. Or better yet, imagine you are meeting this person for a "blind date." What can you do to get to know your date without preconceived ideas about who they are?"

## EROTIC DATES (WEEKLY)

As life becomes complex, we have to set aside time for sex, instead of waiting to be in the mood. Erotic dates are private dates in the bedroom (or another place where sex is possible) to connect physically and emotionally. It is about creating an opportunity to exchange eros energy in any way that appeals to you at the moment.

There are many reasons to engage in sexual activity without craving sex. If you remember the passion pyramid from chapter 5, you know that sex can be about release, bonding, play, or transcendence. Erotic dates can be set up for any one or a combination of these purposes. Moreover, many of us feel aroused *after* sex, which is another reason erotic dates are essential for your eros-sustenance plan.

However, and not uncommonly, couples who have been together for a while lose their spontaneous drive. Newer models of sexuality, particularly for women, recommend that we embrace a concept called "willingness,"[33] which acknowledges the many reasons and many ways we might be sexual together.[34] Stage 3 couples incorporate "willingness" as part of their eros-sustenance plan, whether they crave sex or not.

I suggest that you begin these dates by taking time as a couple to shift states, starting with ten minutes of mindfulness. Few people are ready to have sex immediately after inhabiting other roles. We may need time to off-gas our frustrations of the day, decelerate, or come into a safe connection (see page 207 for ideas).

So, what do we do on our erotic dates?

Before the date, decide how much time you will take for it and whether you are going freestyle or using a structure. Let each other know if anything is off the table in terms of activities or areas of the body. We might sensitively ask our partner questions such as, "Is your herpes flaring right now?" or "Do you have sore knees?" or "Do you have particular aches and pains I should know about?" Instead of worrying that something will go wrong or you will get injured, name it beforehand and decide what kinds of adjustments to make.

Likewise, disclose your limits. When we accept our limits, new paths open up for us. We begin to cautiously explore our edges, knowing we can stop at any time and redirect an experience that is becoming uncomfortable. Erotic stretching is like stretching physically. We can find the "sweet spot" that feels good (albeit edgy) without tearing a muscle.

Your date does not have to include penetration or even involve the genitals. If you are uncomfortable with "having sex," it might help to have a broad menu of activities from which to choose. Your time together might consist of one or a combination of activities such as deep kissing, mindful touch, oral sex, anal play, penetration, ear play (or arm, leg, or toe play), or some version of parts play for a minute to several hours.

Of course, these are only suggestions. Maybe one person wants a sensual foot rub and the other oral sex. We don't have to want the same thing. Moreover, as goal-free sex liberates us from destination tyranny, there is no pressure to get anywhere or complete anything. We can agree to stop after five minutes.

It's a good idea to spend time teaming around designing your dates, especially in the beginning. You might also use a portion of your tending dates (see below) to design a few erotic dates for the future.

Here are some things you might discuss before the date:

Are we taking turns or both engaging at once?

Do we want to do an exercise, like mindful touch?

Do we want to use EROS to practice erotic attunement?

Do we want to practice stop-study-share? What's our word or signal if we're going to pause?

Do we want to be our usual selves or do parts play?

Are we up for planting a heart if we touch into something painful?

Is this for pleasure, healing, or both?

What do we need to do first to come into connection?

Do we want to role-play or go freestyle? (If role-play, do we codesign a scenario or does one of us set it up?)

Do we want to keep our clothes on?

Do we feel like giving one-way? If so, does partner A follow their curiosity, or is partner B going to give partner A direction?

Are we open to penetration if it goes that way?

How important is having an orgasm?

## TENDING DATES (MONTHLY)

Erotic tending dates are a time to share your feelings and thoughts with each other and to reflect on your erotic relationship together. Mindful communication is at the heart of stage 3 relationships. As with the erotic dates, I recommend that you start these dates with ten minutes of mindfulness meditation together. At the end of your mindfulness practice, allow a few minutes for you each to feel into your erotic connection, and see what arises. Notice if there is anything to clear, explore, ask for, or check out with your partner related to sex.

Go back through the "Mindful Activities and Naked Reflections" at the end of each chapter. Better yet, generate your own naked reflections as an activity for one of these dates. If you have been exploring reactions and triggers separately, now is the time to share discoveries from mindful self-study. What are you observing about yourself during sex? What are you curious about within yourself? How does your relational container need tending?

While your conversation will be naked, you want to have your clothes on while you have them. Tending dates are separate from erotic dates. They are for strengthening your relational container, revising contracts and covenants, sharing desires, making a repair, and getting radically naked emotionally.

You can also use these dates for mindful coinvestigation of triggers and aversions (see chapters 3 and 4). Refrain from blaming each other and own your experience. Take seriously your commitment to use the erotic portal for growth and lean into challenges, respectfully and with compassion.

## Dancing with the Sweet Spot of Safety

Lively discourse is underway concerning the importance of safety when it comes to sex. Some researchers frame the discussion by looking at our biology; others concern themselves with the emotional connection between partners; and still others focus on how the brain responds to aversive and arousing stimuli. However, more is not always better when it comes to safety and sex. Too much security puts eros into a stupor.

Viewing the brain as having both a gas and a brake pedal can help you find your sweet spot of sexual safety, explains Emily Negoski, the author of *Come as You Are*.[35] Most of us are aware of the gas pedal—the sexual excitatory system (SES)—which revs up our arousal. It is conditioned to respond to whatever cues and stimuli that we find arousing.

We also have a sexual inhibitory system (SIS, or brake) that inhibits arousal under threat. It responds to concerns about safety, ranging from physical safety to the risk of an unwanted pregnancy or erectile dysfunction to fears of being interrupted by a child. Our SIS can also switch on when we encounter off-putting and unsexy activities, smells, or sensations, such as itchy sheets, animals on the bed, and a photo of our parents on the nightstand. These are clearly not life-threatening, but are definitely PEP-inhibiting and affect our sex lives.

So, while most of us try to get more turned on for sex, Nagoski recommends that we also turn off our turn-offs. Take an inventory of possible brake-pedal inducers: What threats can you minimize? Do you need to make agreements ahead of time to shower and brush your teeth before sex? Do you need to use a more reliable method of birth control or install a lock on your door so your SIS can turn off?

Many of the couples I work with are particularly sensitive to their physical environment. Feng shui experts tell us to rid our bedroom of clutter, choose warm or neutral colors, and add symmetry to our end tables and lamps. How might you create a welcoming environment for eros? What would help you find the right gas-to-brake ratio?

To push on the gas, we have sometimes first to feel safe enough to surrender. Sue Carter, who is the director emerita of the famed Kinsey Institute, believes that sex requires a state of "immobility without fear."[36] In other words, we have to surrender without getting frozen—especially for penetration. The key to establishing this state may be oxytocin, which prevents the dorsal vagal nerve from shutting us down completely.

By now, you've undoubtedly heard that we release oxytocin with orgasm and breastfeeding. Did you also know that we issue this love drug through long hugs, eye contact, sensual touch, and intimate conversation? According to Stephan Porges, these activities may be a kind of neural "love code" for mammals.[37] Oxytocin stimulates our "care and connection" system, which is why you may want to make time for these things before sex.[38] Massage, warm baths, soothing music, and sharing a meal are also oxytocin-enhancing and, therefore, sustenance for eros.

## The Creative Tension of Connected Longing

Let there be spaces in your togetherness,
And let the winds of the heavens dance between you.
—Kahlil Gibran, *The Prophet* [39]

Sex has many paradoxes. The both/and of a mindful approach recognizes that our heart and loins are not always in synch. While some of us push on the gas when we tend to our feelings of emotional attachment and security, others of us lust after the forbidden and risk. Sometimes we want both. Being emotionally naked enables us to establish a safe, intimate connection, which Sue Johnson, the creator of Emotion-Focused Therapy, likens to the music to which we dance.[40] However, we have to watch out that we don't lose the sense of mystery that revs up the gas for most people.

As we saw in chapters 2 and 5, desire and emotional closeness don't go together like a "horse and carriage." For many, passion is born of danger, obstacles, and distance. It grows in stolen moments and forbidden places.[41] While our evolutionary brain experiences closeness as safety, "Eroticism thrives in the space between the self and the other," claims Esther Perel, who has spent her career helping couples reconcile the erotic and the domestic.[42] Nonetheless, many couples (and their therapists) hope that by increasing emotional intimacy, they will eke out more ardor. In most instances, such efforts are futile.

Too much closeness can extinguish the heat of a long-term relationship and exacerbate trance-induced blindness. So, what's the answer? Stage 3 couples find their optimal zone of closeness by establishing a state of "connected longing." Sexual attraction parallels the economics of supply and demand; we put a higher value on things that are hard to come by. Perceived scarcity is a thrill, which is why an upswell in sexual activity can follow war, an affair, illness, and conflict. In that shaky "I don't have you" place, the chase impulse is activated. The other becomes a prized commodity.

To help couples find their optimal zone of closeness, I usually suggest this simple exercise: Bring the palm of either hand just in front of your eyes. Now describe your palm. If you are like most people, your palm will appear as an indiscriminate blur. Now, move your hand back until you can make out the many lines and veins crisscrossing your palm and fingers. Then, move the hand farther out, so the lines become indistinct again. Now, find the position where you can see the lines most clearly. This activity illustrates the sweet spot of connected longing. You can see each other, and there's also space between you.

You might consider whether you and your partner are knitted too close together to experience longing. On the other hand, as a couple, you may be suffering from continental drift. If you are too disconnected, clear whatever is coming between you. Start spending time together and engage in affectionate touch. According to one study, physical affection is the key to staying "madly in love" in a long-term relationship.[43]

Besides adjusting the space between you, you can generate a state of connected longing by remembering that you will not have each other forever. Sooner or later, this journey will end. You can try this reality now by considering how your life would change if your beloved were not in it. What wouldn't you have that you may be taking for granted? This activity can help you recognize the many gifts you may be receiving that you don't see through the eyes of familiarity. Remembering that we are on borrowed time can help us release old hurts, choose our battles carefully, and accept our partner's quirks.

## Keep a Light on for Me: Solo Erotic Sustenance

Erotic Sustenance is a couple's project, but it also requires some solo play. Both partners need to keep their pilot light lit whether or not they are engaging in partner sex. The truth is that we are responsible for maintaining a connection to eros independent of our partner's desire and efforts to seduce and arouse us. Moreover, an inside-out orientation to pleasure begins with us. We kindle eros energy separately; then shine it on the other.

Your personal eros-sustenance plan may include embodiment practices, imagery exercises, physical activity, mindfulness, and self-pleasuring. You can start by experiencing your body as the conduit of eros energy and savoring moments of sensual pleasure inside and outside of you. Befriend your fantasies and linger with erotic impulses or feelings, whether they lead to partner sex or not. Engage in daily acts of sensuality that feed your body. For instance, notice the feel of soft fabric against your skin, the taste of nourishing or exotic food flavors, the shape of a tree, the sound of the wind, a bird chirping or a soulful piece of music. Eros is in all of those places. It is waiting for you.

## Tending the Mind: The Superfood of Our Eros-Sustenance Plan

As we've seen, great sex is born of both a state of mind that is curious and exploratory and a body that is sensitive, responsive, and attuned. Mindfulness supports all of these things and improves sexual satisfaction,[44] which is why it is the hub of Passion and Presence (see figure 7.2, "Mindfulness Hub").

In terms of sustenance, we might think of mindfulness as an essential building block of our erotic practice, which is why I recommend that you meditate daily. Meditating before having sex can enliven the eros-enhancing states of presence, curiosity, and sensitivity, and with time, consolidate them into more permanent traits. So, when couples practice mindfulness as an erotic team, their relationships become more satisfying and stable.[45]

Consider bringing these elements of mindfulness to your eros-sustenance plan:

**Presence.** We can't underestimate the power of presence to enliven a relationship. As John Welwood says, "In love's early stages, powerful qualities of our being—openness, peace, expansiveness, delight—simply emerge, unbidden, out of the heightened sense of presence we experience with our partner."[46] While these qualities initially come from the prick of Cupid's golden arrow, at stage 3 we can

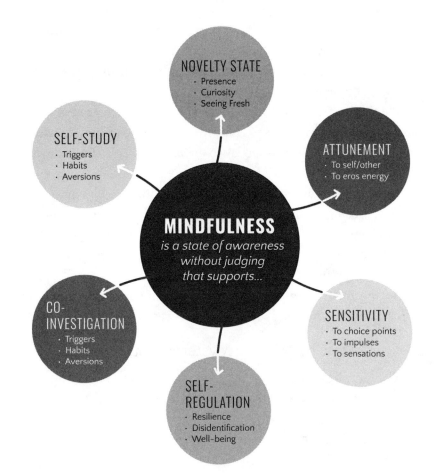

**FIGURE 7.2 MINDFULNESS HUB**

The Mindfulness Hub illustrates how all of the passionate and present skills
grow out of mindfulness and a mindful mind-set.

cultivate presence through mindfulness and an intention to remain
enchanted lifelong.

**Acceptance, empathy, and nonjudgment.** Mindful couples are
better able to take the other's point of view and are less blaming and
rigid in their judgments of their partner. They can accept their partner
as they are, instead of investing tremendous amounts of energy in trying
to change the other.[47]

**Resilience after conflict.** A huge boon to our relationships is the
ability to address conflict effectively. Mindful couples bounce back

more quickly after arguments.[48] They get over arguments without hanging onto anger or bearing grudges. As mentioned earlier, they produce less cortisol during conflicts, which helps them stay regulated throughout disagreements.[49]

**Flexibility.** One aspect of a good relationship is that it can adjust to change. Mindfulness seems to cultivate resilience to the only constant in life—change. We are also likely to update our views of our partner over time and across multiple contexts.[50]

**Happiness.** Many studies show that mindfulness enhances personal well-being and individual happiness.[51] Happiness contributes to relationship health and satisfaction, as well. Why not give yourselves the best possible chance of being in good states together by establishing a regular mindfulness practice?

**Seeing-fresh mind-set.** Perhaps the most important element of all is that a mindful mind-set supports novelty seeking during sex.[52]

## Making Magic by Meeting Mystery: Erotic Alchemy

The most beautiful experience we can have is the mysterious. Whoever does not know it and can no longer wonder, no longer marvel, is as good as dead.
—Albert Einstein[53]

When it comes to quality partner sex, I believe that the people involved and their states of mind are more important than techniques or specific activities. If this is the case, then how can we work with our consciousness to stay curious and open to our partner in the face of familiarity? The fact is that people become boring to us only when we fix them in our mind's eye. While we see our reality as seamless and unchanging, this idea is a "controlled hallucination," claims Michael Pollan, the author of *How to Change Your Mind*.[54]

Many researchers believe that we manufacture our reality from our sense data and the models in our memories—a process that scientists call predictive coding.[55] I call it trance-blindness.

So, what *is* real? We live in an emergent universe where everything, including ourselves and our partner, is in continuous flux. There is no enduring self or central order except in our minds. Facing this truth can be exciting, frightening, and challenging. "Uncertainty is a complex brain's biggest challenge, and predictive coding evolved to help us reduce it," says Pollan.[56] If something looks familiar, we make quick but often inaccurate judgments about what it is based on our inner models derived from previous experiences and judgments.

Scientists call the parts of our brain that account for our tendency to default to well-worn mental routes the default mode network (DMN). The DMN takes us to the same places again and again—in our minds. We ruminate, make predictions about the future, reflect on ourselves and our partner, missing out on the ever-changing now. All of this mind wandering generates states of mind that are neither sexy nor happy.[57]

The DMN also regulates what comes into our consciousness. We become trapped in habitual modes of thought that create not only states of mood but also perceptual biases that limit what we can experience.[58] Children presumably don't have such a system until around age nine; which may explain why they are so easily awed.[59] We lose our awe when we become "know-it-alls." Unfortunately, our ways of thinking and perceiving become only more fixed as we age—unless we keep the windows of perception open and limber.

If so many "truths" are fixed only in our minds, then how can we keep our mind open? How can we maintain an open, not-knowing, ready-to-be-awed headspace for magical sex over the long haul? We have to watch out for beliefs like "I'm too old for sex," "There's nothing new for us to experience as a couple," "It won't be very good," or other well-worn expectations that bar us from making magic together.

Mindfulness offers a way out of this prison since it helps us enter a much larger room of our mind. We can resist "shrinking by thinking" and open up to a broader living reality that comes into focus when we disidentify from our thoughts, feelings, and perceptions and see fresh.

Numerous studies show reduced activity in the DMN during meditation.[60] Regular meditators also have less DMN activity even when they are not meditating, presumably because they are in the moment more.[61] Not only does mindfulness train us to be present during sex, but mindful sex may itself be a gateway to an expanded consciousness. For when we are fully engaged in the present, the DMN goes nearly still. In the open plane of possibility or pure erotic potential, we can see, feel, and touch anew. When we embark on the naked path in this way, our potential for pleasure—and awe—is enormous.

"How vast is the landscape of sexual pleasure? More vast than we know, for much of it remains untapped," claimed the late Gina Ogden, a pioneer of modern sex therapy and the author of *The Heart and Soul of Sex*. "It lies in the realm of ecstasy, mystery, and magic, the realm where all paths flow into a unified whole."[62] Mindful sex takes us to the liminal spaces between the fully formed outlines of ordinary waking consciousness and the "petite mort," or little death of orgasm. Here is where animal and divine drink from the same river. However, when passion becomes tarnished, and we succumb to numbing routines, that magical zone becomes harder to locate.

It is when we drop our templates and meet fresh, that we find it again. We discover that we—and our beloved—are not as stable or fixed as appears. Something nascent and unknown—possibly unknowable—takes place at this magical watering hole. As Michael Ventura says, "In the shape-shifting qualities of deep sexuality, change is ever-present; it can even be said that in the throes of such sex, sex is change."[63]

The transformative power of eros is manifest when we enter sex through one door and come out through another—changed. Exchanging eros energy thus has the potential to transform both parties into something new. The alchemy of eros is the mystery of the dark: the creative core of emergence. It is where we discover and also become "other things." There are certainly other means to "open the doors" of perception. However, sex got you here on the planet and most likely drew you together as a couple. Perhaps, now, it can be a springboard to higher consciousness and transformation in the fullest sense, as in erotic alchemy.

We end our journey here at erotic sustenance. No longer a victim of the golden or leaden arrows, we awaken to our erotic potential with a vision that fits our changing desires and capacities. The naked path is ultimately a journey of transformation, discovery, and awe. Along the way, we encounter great beauty, even magic, as well as disappointment and loss. As Diane Ackerman says: "It began in mystery, and it will end in mystery, but what a savage and beautiful country lies in between."[64] Whether you choose to stay on the naked path or veer off from here, I know your trip will be full of both light and shadow. May the illuminating power of eros guide your way.

## MINDFUL ACTIVITIES AND NAKED REFLECTIONS

. . . . . . . . . . . . . . . . . . . . . . . . . . . . . . . . . . . . . . . . . . . . . . . . . . . .

## Crafting Our Sustenance Plan

. . . . . . . . . . . . . . . . . . . . . . . . . . . . . . . . . . . . . . . . . . . . . . . . . . . .

Consider crafting your plan on a self-guided "couple's retreat," or you can do each part separately during your erotic tending dates. If you decide to break up the activity, schedule when you will do parts 2, 3, and 4 now rather than leaving it up to chance.

### Part 1: The Elements of Your Plan

Sit down together and spend five to ten minutes in mindfulness. Then, go back through the chapter, section by section, to see what applies to you. How do you want to tend your erotic life individually and as a couple? What kind of magic do you need to make right now?

Does your physical body or self-image need tending?

How can you find your sweet spots of safety, arousal, and connection?

Does your definition of sex and eros need to expand?

What are you each willing to do to stay in a state of erotic awe?

### Part 2: Crafting Your Plan

Once you've answered these questions, explore the kind of eros-sustenance plan that makes sense for you in this season of your life. Be as specific as possible, and list everything that occurs to each of you. Decide whether or not to put this into a covenant.

## Part 3: Exploring Barriers

Take turns answering the following questions in mindfulness.

Partner A gets mindful first. Then, partner B asks partner A the first question.

Partner A will wait for an answer to well up from inside rather than going with a quick response. When the answer comes, partner A shares. Partner B writes down the answer.

Go through all the questions with partner A before switching to B or switch roles after answering the first two questions.

What are some internal barriers you are likely to face that might get in the way of implementing our plan? How can we work with these barriers?

What might motivate you to be "willing" to have sex, even when your body doesn't crave it? How can I gently remind you of this when I/we are avoiding sex?

## Part 4: Fun and Romance, Erotic, and Tending Dates

Schedule your three kinds of dates for three months out. Come up with a list of activities you might do together for your fun and romance dates. Then, plan your first erotic date by going through the questions on pages 205–206.

# Acknowledgments

Historians tell us the social landscape is changing.[1] While we still have a ways to go to bridge the gender gap, we've thankfully scratched the word "obey" from our marriage vocabulary. Moreover, in the Western world, most women no longer need to marry for survival, land rights, or children. Without the binding force of traditional roles and mandates, is there any reason to establish a long-term relationship nowadays?

No other writer addressed this question with as much poetic dash as the late John Welwood, who said yes, but not for sentimental reasons. Even romance has limitations. Instead, he claimed that relationships could serve a sacred purpose, which is to heal the wound to our hearts. He alleged that this wound is the source of our lovesickness and many other afflictions. We feel undeserving of love and push it away. In so doing, we close off to life and ourselves.

I believe the same holds for our sexuality; we feel ashamed of our desires and undeserving of pleasure. I developed Passion and Presence to help couples heal their "eros wound" and grow through their sexual journey together. Awakened intimacy is ultimately a way to open to ourselves, each other, and also to life.

This book pays homage to Welwood, in particular, and other luminaries on conscious relationships, such as Gay and Kathryn Hendricks and Jett Psaris and Marlena Lyons. Thank you for lighting the path and placing signposts for me to carry your pioneering legacy into the sexual arena.

As a psychologist, Welwood recognized the danger of "spiritual bypassing," where we use self-transcendence to skirt the shadowy dark emotions that cloud our capacity to love. If we don't shine a light on the dark corners of our emotional life, our goodwill will dissolve into reactivity whenever we are triggered. It is for this reason that couples need skills to tolerate the feelings that arise when they get naked with each other.

In developing the skill set of Passion and Presence, I borrowed liberally from Hakomi Mindful Somatic Psychotherapy. This Eastern-infused body psychotherapy rests on the tenets of complexity theory and incorporates advances in neuroscience, trauma recovery, and attachment theory. I have been rewarded many times over as a Hakomi trainer. For this, I must firstly thank Ron Kurtz, the founder of Hakomi, who, along with my other original teacher, Jon Eisman, put me on a path that has been the centerpiece of my professional life since 1985.

Also, my colleagues Rob Fisher, Jaci Hull, and Halko Weiss have enlarged my understanding of working with couples tremendously. However, the entire Hakomi faculty has inspired my passion and presence, with special thanks to the Matrix team.

Halko Weiss, the creator of Hakomi Embodied and Aware Relationship Training (HEART), graciously allowed me to take his reciprocal interaction loop and associated skills and repackage them in accord with my language and model. With his blessings, I've borrowed many of HEART's core concepts in chapter 3, "Erotic Cooperation."

I also want to thank Cedar Barstow, the founder of the Right Use of Power Institute, for permitting me to use her term *response-agility* to describe a core feature of stage 3 erotic coupling.

Many of my ideas on the performance trance evolved from a workshop I presented in 2006 with Melissa Grace called "Falling in Love with Your Imperfect Self." Melissa coined the term "the Olympian imperative" found in chapter 2.

My views on trance states come primarily from Tara Brach, Arthur Deikman, Charles Tart, and Stephen Wolinsky. I also want to acknowledge Jon Eisman for his elegant articulation of trance states in his work, Recreation of the Self. My gratitude goes to Richard Schwartz, the creator of Internal Family Systems, for supporting my work and allowing me to quote liberally from his article "Revealing Our Many Selves in the

Bedroom." The Internal Family Systems model informs some critical concepts of chapters 3 and 5.

My appreciation also goes to my outstanding Somatic Experiencing instructor, Diane Poole Heller. Somatic Experiencing is a method for healing trauma developed by Peter Levine that informs the detaching process I use with Sue and Barney.

The wisdom, vision, and practical know-how of many sexperts inform this text: Patti Britton, Rosalyn Dischiavo, Suzanne Iasenza, Ian Kerner, Marty Klein, Joe Kort, Barry McCarthy, Tammy Nelson, Gina Ogden, Esther Perel, David Schnarch, and William Stayton—to name a few. In particular, I would like to thank Tammy Nelson. I was spellbound the first time I heard her speak, and I continue to steep in Tammy's wisdom, humor, and practical ways of enlivening eros in long-term relationships.

Likewise, I was hooked when I heard Esther Perel apply the term "poetics" to sex in 2009. Few people have explored the perils and possibilities of postmodern love so compellingly. I've integrated many of her ideas in Passion and Presence. David Schnarch needs a special mention also for asserting from the get-go that erotic challenges are catalysts for growth.

The late Gina Ogden was the author of thirteen books and a pioneer in sexology. She was among the first to emphasize pleasure over performance. A generous-hearted champion for newcomers like me, Gina encouraged Chelsea Wakefield to attend a talk that I gave at the Grove Park Inn in Asheville, North Carolina, in 2013. This chance meeting was pivotal in my decision to follow through on becoming certified as a sex therapist. Chelsea is the author of *In Search of Aphrodite*, and creator of the Luminous Woman workshops. A luminous woman herself, I look forward to our cross-pollination in the years to come.

As for the writing, I flanked myself with two remarkable thought partners and editors, Dido Clark and Kathleen Gregory. Dido helped me hone my message years ago and joined forces with me in structuring this book. She graciously handled the details of the project and gently oriented me when I got lost in my big ideas. Kathleen Gregory signed me with Shambhala, so I was crestfallen when she left the company soon after. Three months before I submitted my manuscript, I tracked down Kathleen and asked her to bring her editing chops to my project. To my delight, she agreed. These two women were the polishing cloth that made my book sparkle.

I also want to acknowledge my friend and original writing buddy, Kathy Brown. Kathy gave me honest feedback and companionship in the isolating bubble that writers gleefully retreat into to incubate their ideas, and subsequently feel interned by when their words aren't flowing.

An unforgettable moment was receiving an email from Stephan Downes, the contracts manager at Shambhala Publications, that said: "Welcome to the Shambhala family." Words cannot express how proud I am to join your family. Sarah Stanton, my editor at Shambhala, and her editing assistant, Samantha Ripley, have been a delight to work with and helped me smooth the remaining crinkles out of the text.

Thank you, Julia Corley, for your graceful, gracious involvement with Passion and Presence and for introducing me to our brilliant graphic designer, Linda Misiura. Linda did the visual branding for Passion and Presence retreats and created the figures for *Passion and Presence*. If a picture is worth a thousand words, yours speak a million. It was after I sent my images to the publisher that Kathleen wrote, "The diagrams give me a much deeper appreciation for your model and how beneficial it is."

The transformational journey I've been on with my dearest friends, Lyn and Tony, and my deep-dive group, helps me trust the naked path even more. With you, I've taken down all the masks, and the love keeps on flowing. Thanks to Jean, Lore, and Melissa for holding me in your hearts and for holding my hand when I've been shaky.

Halko—my erotic team—you've taught me so much about love. Thank you for choosing me and telling me daily that "I am The One." This book would not have come into being without your gentle and firm insistence to "write your book," and believing, without a shadow of a doubt, that I had something of value to offer. Thanks for being so naked with me as a partner, and generously tolerating my long exile from our life together so I could take care of my mom and wrap up this project. Thanks even more for opening your arms—wide—each time I return from my exploits and running home to me after yours. Our journey together as partners, lovers, and colleagues is full of surprises and unanticipated adventures.

To my amazing clients and the couples who have taken our retreats, thank you for letting me tag along on your journey. You have no idea how many gifts I receive from knowing you. Often enough, you are my teachers and not the other way around. I want to send a special shout out to the participants of our retreats and my Hakomi students, who time and again have asked me, "When is your book coming out?" The answer is now!

# Glossary

**awakened intimacy**  Using the erotic portal for awareness, growth, and transformation.

**black light syndrome**  When early imprints switch on during sexual activity, and old wounds light up at the same time.

**both/and approach**  Using sex for *both* pleasure *and* healing.

**care cycle**  Using the three R's (i.e., reveal, reach, and repair) to build a collaborative and compassionate alliance.

**compassionate contact**  Feeling into your partner's hidden, protected state and guessing what they might be feeling beneath their protector. Naming your guess in a caring way.

**eros energy**  Life-force energy that vitalizes us and turns us on. Similar terms may be *drive, libido,* and *creative spark.*

**erotic attunement**  Using your felt sense to connect to eros energy individually and as a couple, and keying off of this energy in an unscripted call-and-response.

**imprint portfolio**  A collection of experiences we encode/file outside of awareness.

**interoception**  The ability to detect sensations and internal signals from the body.

**legacy state**  When the feelings of helplessness, fear, and pain we felt as children are restimulated in the present.

**mindful coinvestigation**  A co-constructed experiment to explore an unpleasant feeling, sensation, or reaction. For the research, partner A provides the trigger (or stimulus), so partner B can mindfully study what occurs automatically in response.

**mindful self-study** Turning inward and directing attention to a present felt experience, so feelings, sensations, images, memories, and beliefs surface from the bottom-up.

**mindful sex** Sex where the inner observer has open eyes; a quality of presence and attention during sex that is curious and allowing.

**naked path** Consciously working with barriers to your pure erotic potential that become visible in a long-term relationship.

**novelty state** Staying curious in the face of familiarity to discover something new.

**parts play** Letting usually hidden internal parts have a place in your erotic "us" zone.

**planting a heart** Receiving and encoding a corrective experience provided by your partner to transform a sexual wound from the past.

**pure erotic potential (PEP)** The unlimited creativity available when we drop goals, reference points, habits, filters, and expectations and meet with an "anything is possible" state of mind.

**radical nakedness** Being emotionally unprotected with your partner by revealing inner experiences that are usually hidden by your "protectors."

**reciprocal interaction loop (RIL)** A stuck reinforcing interaction between each partner's "protector" states/parts that occurs when their legacy states are triggered.

**seeing fresh (touching fresh, meeting fresh)** Seeing anew what you have seen many times before to avoid falling into habitual modes of perceiving and experiencing.

**somatic self-attunement** Using your interoception or "felt sense" to determine whether to go toward or decline a sexual activity.

**stage 3 erotic coupling (re-enchantment)** Making a commitment to practice awakened intimacy, or conscious erotic coupling. It requires a willingness to be vulnerable, a set of mindfulness-based skills, and a solid alliance as a couple.

**trance** Being identified with a narrow and distorted view of reality that we take as the "truth."

# Notes

## INTRODUCTION

1. *Passion & Presence*® retreats are trademarked. To learn more, go to www .passionandpresence.com.
2. Maryam Sanati, "Sexless Marriage," *Today's Parent* (blog), January 10, 2011, www.todaysparent.com/family/sexless-marriage/.
3. Gay Hendricks and Kathlyn Hendricks, *Conscious Loving: The Journey to Co-commitment* (New York: Bantam, 1992), 43.

## CHAPTER 1: AWAKENED INTIMACY

1. www.brainyquote.com/quotes/h_l_mencken_143434.
2. Michael Liebowitz, *The Chemistry of Love* (New York: Berkley Books, 1983).
3. Helen Fisher, *Why We Love: The Nature and Chemistry of Romantic Love* (New York: Owl Books Henry Holt, 2004).
4. Robert Kegan, *In Over Our Heads: The Mental Demands of Modern Life* (Cambridge, MA: Harvard College, 1994).
5. Lisa Dawn Hamilton and Cindy M. Meston, "Chronic Stress and Sexual Arousal," *The Journal of Sexual Medicine*, 10 (2013): 2443–54, doi:10.1111 /jsm.12249.
6. Naomi Wolf, *Vagina* (New York: Harper Collins, 2013); Susan Johnson, "Why Emotional Safety is the Defining Feature of Good Sex," *Psychotherapy Networker* (blog), no date, www.psychotherapynetworker.org/blog /details/783/why-emotional-safety-is-the-defining-feature-of-good; Bethy Squires, "Why Some Women Don't Feel Pleasure During Sex," *Vice* (blog), August 29, 2016, www.vice.com/en_us/article/wjeq3b/why-some-women-dont-feel-pleasure-during-sex.
7. Fisher, *Why We Love.*

8. Katherine Wu, "Love, Actually: The Science Behind Lust, Attraction, and Companionship," *Harvard University: The Graduate School of Arts and Sciences* (blog), February 14, 2017, http://sitn.hms.harvard.edu/flash/2017/love-actually-science-behind-lust-attraction-companionship/.

9. Dan Savage, *Savage Love: Straight Answers from America's Most Popular Sex Columnist* (New York: Penguin Books, 1998).

10. www.brainyquote.com/quotes/dee_hock_285469.

11. William Shakespeare, *Sonnet 137*, lines 1–2. www.shakespeares-sonnets.com/sonnet/137.

12. Margaret Mahler, Fred Pine, and Anni Bergman, *The Psychological Birth of the Human Infant: Symbiosis and Individuation* (New York: Basic Books, 2008).

13. Anonymous.

14. Marnia Robinson, *Cupid's Poisoned Arrow: From Habit to Harmony in Sexual Relationships* (Berkeley, CA: North Atlantic Books, 2009).

15. Anaïs Nin, *The Diary of Anaïs Nin, Vol. 3: 1939–1944*, ed. Gunther Stuhlmann (New York: Harcourt Brace Jovanovich), 168.

16. John Welwood, *Journey of the Heart: The Path of Conscious Love* (New York: Harper Perennial), 13.

17. John Welwood, *Perfect Love, Imperfect Relationships: Healing the Wound of the Heart* (Boston, MA: Shambhala Publications, 2007); John Welwood, "Absolute and Relative Love," 2006, www.johnwelwood.com/articles/Absolute_and_Relative_Love.pdf.

18. Marion F. Solomon, *Narcissism and Intimacy: Love and Marriage in an Age of Confusion* (New York and London: W. W. Norton), 40.

19. Miriam Greenspan, *Healing through the Dark Emotions: The Wisdom of Grief, Fear, and Despair* (Boston, MA: Shambhala, 2003), 93.

20. Kahlil Gibran, "On Love," in *The Prophet* (New York: Alfred A. Knopf, 1994), 12.

21. In complexity theory, the triggering event is called a *perturbation*. For more details, see www.calresco.org/perturb.htm.

22. Anaïs Nin, *The Diary of Anaïs Nin, Vol. 1: 1931–1934* (New York: Harcourt Brace Jovanovich, 1969).

23. Daniel Siegel, *Aware: The Science and Practice of Presence, the Groundbreaking Meditation Practice* (New York: Penguin Random House, 2018).

24. Charles Tart, *Waking Up: Overcoming the Obstacles to Human Potential* (Boston, MA: New Science Library, 1986).

25. Arthur Deikman, *The Observing Self: Mysticism and Psychotherapy* (Boston, MA: Beacon Press, 1983).

26. Maryann Camaroto, public talk, San Francisco, 2016.

27. Welwood, *Journey of the Heart*, 13.

## CHAPTER 2: EROTIC PRESENCE

1. Michael Michalko, "Change the Way You Look at Things and the Things You Look at Change," *The Creativity Post* (blog), July 11, 2012, www.creativitypost .com/article/change_the_way_you_look_at_things_and_the_things_you_ look_at_change.

2. Thomas Lewis, Fari Amini, and Richard Lannon, *A General Theory of Love* (New York: Vintage Books/Random House, 2000); Kendra Cherry, "How Confirmation Bias Works," *Verywellmind*, (blog) November 27, 2019, www .verywellmind.com/what-is-a-confirmation-bias-2795024; Mohsen Rafiei et al., "Optimizing Perception: Attended and Ignored Stimuli Create Opposing Perceptual Biases," *PsyArXiv* (September 26, 2019), doi:10.31234/ osf.io/m79nu.

3. Benjamin Scheibehenne, Jutta Mata, and Peter Todd, "Older but Not Wiser—Predicting a Partner's Preferences Gets Worse with Age," *Journal of Consumer Psychology* 21, no. 2 (March 2011): 184–91, doi:10.1016/j .jcps.2010.08.001.

4. Annie Murphy Paul, "Mind Reading," *Psychology Today* (blog), September 1, 2007, www.psychologytoday.com/us/articles/200709/mind-reading.

5. Anne Fischer, "The Role of Core Organizing Beliefs in Hakomi Therapy," in *Hakomi Mindfulness-Centered Somatic Psychotherapy*, eds. Halko Weiss, Greg Johanson, and Lorena Monda (New York: Norton, 2015), 66–75; Daniel Siegel, *Aware*.

6. Noah Rasheta, "The Three Poisons," episode 91, *Secular Buddhism Podcast*, February 3, 2019, https://secularbuddhism.com/91-the-three-poisons/.

7. Vivia Chen, "There's a Bit of Gabe MacConaill in All of Us," *New York Law Journal* (blog), November 15, 2018, www.law.com/newyorklaw journal/2018/11/15/theres-a-bit-of-gabe-macconaill-in-all-of-us/?slre turn=20190520081853.

8. Peggy Orenstein, *Girls and Sex: Navigating the Complicated New Landscape* (New York: HarperCollins, 2016).

9. Noah Rasheta, "The Three Poisons."

10. Thich Nhat Hanh, "Dharma Talk: Transforming Negative Habit Energies," *Mindfulnessbell* (blog), December 2015, www.mindfulnessbell.org /archive/2015/12/dharma-talk-transforming-negative-habit-energies; Pema Chodron, *Taking the Leap: Freeing Ourselves from Old Habits and Fears* (Boulder, CO: Shambhala, 2010).

11. Liz Hall, "How Practicing Mindfulness in the Workplace Can Boost Productivity," *Occupational Health & Wellbeing* (blog), May 1, 2013, www.personneltoday.com/hr/how-practising-mindfulness-in-the-workplace-can-boost-productivity/#.Uh3TvWTXgzE.

12. Matt Mattei, "Anderson Cooper: How a Story on Mindful Living Transformed His Life," *Meetmindful* (blog), www.meetmindful.com/anderson-cooper-how-a-story-on-mindful-living-transformed-his-life/; Susan Minuk, "Dan Harris: Exploring Mindfulness as the New Superpower," *Canadian Jewish News* (blog), June 21, 2019, www.cjnews.com/perspectives/features/dan-harris-exploring-mindfulness-new-superpower; Dan Harris, *Meditation for Fidgety Skeptics: A 10% Happier How-to Book* (New York: Spiegel & Grau, 2018).

13. Jeffrey M. Greeson, "Mindfulness Research Update: 2008," *Complementary Health Practice Review* 14, no. 1 (January 2009): 10–18, doi:10.1177/1533210108329862; Mark G. Williams and Jon Kabat-Zinn, "Mindfulness: Diverse Perspectives on its Meaning, Origins, and Multiple Applications at the Intersection of Science and Dharma," *Contemporary Buddhism* 12, no. 1 (June 14, 2011): 1–18, doi:10.1080/14639947.2011.564811; Daphne David and Jeffrey Hayes, "What Are the Benefits of Mindfulness? A Practice Review of Psychotherapy-Related Research," *Psychotherapy Theory Research Practice Training* 48, no. 2 (June 2011): 198–208, doi:10.1037/a0022062.

14. Tainya C. Clarke et al., "Trends in the Use of Complementary Health Approaches among Adults: United States, 2002–2012." *National Health Statistics Reports*, no 79 (Hyattsville, MD: National Center for Health Statistics), 2015, https://nccih.nih.gov/research/statistics/NHIS/2012/mind-body/meditation; Amy Norton, "Number of Americans Practicing Yoga, Meditation Surged in Last Six Years," *UPI* (blog), November 8, 2018, www.upi.com/Health_News/2018/11/08/Number-of-Americans-practicing-yoga-meditation-surged-in-last-six-years/4871541738659/.

15. Joan Sutherland, "What Is Enlightenment?" *Lion's Roar* (blog), December 19, 2015, https://www.lionsroar.com/what-is-enlightenment/.

16. Charles Tart, *Waking Up: Overcoming the Obstacles to Human Potential* (Lincoln, NE: iUniverse, 2001).

17. Jon Eisman, "Categories of Psychological Wounding, Neural Patterns, and Treatment Approaches," *Hakomi Forum* 14–15 (2005): 43–50; Stephen Wolinsky, *Waking From the Trance: A Practical Course for Developing Multi-Dimensional Awareness* (Boulder, CO: Sounds True).

18. Steven Stosney, "Blue-Collar Therapy: The Nitty-Gritty of Lasting Change," *Psychotherapy Networker* (blog) November/December 2013; Wendy Wood,

*Good Habits, Bad Habits: The Science of Making Positive Changes That Stick* (New York: Farrar, Straus and Giroux, 2019).

19. Tara Healey, "Train Your Mind to Work Smarter," *Mindful* (blog), January 31, 2019, www.mindful.org/putting-mindfulness-to-work/.

20. Barry W. McCarthy, "Synchronous and Asynchronous Sexual Experiences: Embrace Each Other's Differences," *Psychology Today* (blog), December 2, 2014, www.psychologytoday.com/us/blog/whats-your-sexual-style/201412 /synchronous-and-asynchronous-sexual-experiences.

21. Sengstan, *Hsin Hsin Ming,* "Verse on the Faith Mind," in *Teachings of the Buddha,* ed. Jack Kornfield (Boston, MA: Shambhala Publications, 1993), 144.

22. Ellen Langer, *Mindfulness* (Philadelphia, PA: Merloyd Lawrence Books, 2014).

23. Eugene Gendlin, *Focusing* (New York: Bantam Books/Random House, 1978/2007); Amanda Morin, "Interoception and Sensory Processing Issues: What You Need to Know," *Understood* (blog), www.understood .org/en/learning-attention-issues/child-learning-disabilities/sensory- processing-issues/interoception-and-sensory-processing-issues-what- you-need-to-know.

24. Ariel Handy and Cindy Meston, "Interoception and Awareness of Physi- ological Sexual Arousal in Women with Sexual Arousal Concerns," *Journal of Sex & Marital Therapy* 44, no. 4 (May 19, 2018): 398–409, doi:10.1080/00 92623X.2017.1405305.

25. Marsha Lucas, "Better Sex?" *Mindful* (blog) May 11, 2011, www.mindful .org/better-sex-through-mindfulness-meditation/.

26. Sara Lazar et al., "Meditation Experience Is Associated with Increased Cortical Thickness," *Neuroreport* 16, no. 17 (2005): 1893–97.

27. Stephanie Ortigue, Scott T. Grafton, and Francesco Bianchi-Demicheli, "Correlation Between Insula Activation and Self-Reported Quality of Or- gasm in Women," *NeuroImage* 37 (2007): 551–60.

28. Lori Brotto, *Better Sex Through Mindfulness: How Women Can Cultivate Desire* (Vancouver/Berkeley: Greystone Books, 2018).

29. Jeffrey M. Schwartz and Sharon Begley, *The Mind and the Brain: Neuroplas- ticity and the Power of Mental Force* (New York: ReganBooks/HarperCollins, 2002).

30. Lori A. Brotto et al., "Mindfulness-Based Sex Therapy Improves Genital- Subjective Arousal Concordance in Women with Sexual Desire/Arousal Difficulties," *Archives of Sexual Behavior* 45, no. 8 (2016), 1907–21, https:// doi.org/10.1007/s10508-015-0689-8; Meredith Chivers, "A Brief Update on the Specificity of Sexual Arousal," *Sexual and Relationship Therapy*

25, no. 4 (2010), 407–14, doi:10.1080/14681994.2010.495979; Julia Velten et al., "Investigating Female Sexual Concordance: Do Sexual Excitation and Sexual Inhibition Moderate the Agreement of Genital and Subjective Sexual Arousal in Women?" *Archives of Sexual Behavior* 45, no. 8 (2016): 1957–71, doi:10.1007/s10508-016-0774-7; Kelly D. Suschinsky et al., "The Relationship Between Sexual Functioning and Sexual Concordance in Women," *Journal of Sex & Marital Therapy* 45, no. 3 (2019): doi:10.1080/00 92623X.2018.1518881.

31. Julia Velten and Lori Brotto, "Interoception and Sexual Response in Women with Low Sexual Desire," *PLoS ONE* 12, no. 10 (2017): e0185979, https://doi. org/10.1371/journal.pone.0185979.

32. Pema Chödrön, *The Places That Scare You* (Boston, MA: Shambhala, 2001), 25.

33. T. Flint Sparks, "Assisted Self-Study: Observing the Organization of Experience," in *Hakomi Mindfulness-Centered Somatic Psychotherapy*, eds. Halko Weiss, Greg Johanson, and Lorena Monda (New York: Norton, 2015), 58–65.

34. Barry McCarthy and Lana Wald, "Mindfulness and Good Enough Sex," *Sexual & Relationship Therapy* 28 (2013), https://doi.org/10.1080/14681994 .2013.770829.

35. Coined by Melissa Grace, personal communication 2005.

36. David Neal, Wendy Wood, and Aimee Drolet, "How Do People Adhere to Goals When Willpower Is Low? The Profits (and Pitfalls) of Strong Habits," *Journal of Personality and Social Psychology* 104, no. 6 (June 2013): 959–75.

37. Wayne Dyer, www.goodreads.com/author/quotes/2960.Wayne_W_ Dyer?page=18.

38. Greg Johanson, "Artistic Inspirations: False Colors," *The Annals of the American Psychotherapy Association* 11, no. 3 (2008): 28.

## CHAPTER 3: EROTIC COOPERATION

1. Welwood, *Perfect Love, Imperfect Relationships*, 35.

2. John Welwood, *Love and Awakening: Discovering the Sacred Path of Intimate Relationship* (New York: HarperPerennial, 1996), 7.

3. Carl Rogers, *On Becoming a Person: A Therapist's View of Psychotherapy* (Boston, MA: Houghton Mifflin), 122.

4. Stan Tatkin, *Wired for Love: How Understanding Your Partner's Brain and Attachment Style Can Help You Defuse Conflict and Build a Secure Relationship* (Oakland, CA: New Harbinger Publications, 2011).

5. Daniel Siegel, *The Developing Mind: How Relationships and the Brain Interact to Shape Who We Are* (New York: Guilford Press, 1999), 188.

6. Daniel Siegel, *The Mindful Brain: Reflection and Attunement in the Cultivation of Well-Being* (New York: W. W. Norton, 2007), 314.

7. Cameron Crowe, James L. Brooks, Laurence Mark, Richard Sakai, *Jerry McGuire*. Directed by Cameron Crowe, Sony Pictures Releasing, Culver City, CA, 1996.

8. Jellaludin Rumi, "The Guest House," in *The Essential Rumi*, trans. Coleman Barks, (New York: HarperCollins, 1995), 108.

9. Elaine Hatfield, John Cacioppo, and Richard L. Rapson, "Emotional Contagion," *Current Directions in Psychological Science 2,* no. 3 (June 1993): 96–99, ep10770953, doi:10.1111/1467-8721; Sherrie Bourg Carter, "The Emotional Contagion Scale. How Susceptible Are You to Catching a Bad Case of Emotions?" *Psychology Today* (blog), October 20, 2012, www.psychologytoday.com/us/blog/high-octane-women/201210/the-emotional-contagion-scale.

10. Rainer Maria Rilke, *Letters to a Young Poet*, trans. H. D. Herter (New York and London: W. W. Norton, 1993), 27.

11. David Schnarch, *Passionate Marriage: Keeping Love and Intimacy Alive in Committed Relationships* (New York: W. W. Norton, 2009).

12. Norbert Wiener, *Cybernetics or Control and Communication in the Animal and the Machine* (Cambridge, MA: MIT Press, 1948).

13. Sue Johnson, *Hold Me Tight: Seven Conversations for a Lifetime of Love* (New York: Little, Brown and Company, 2008).

14. Terrence Real, *The New Rules of Marriage: What You Need to Know to Make Love Work* (New York: Ballantine Books, 2007).

15. John Gottman, *The Seven Principles for Making Marriage Work* (New York: Crown, 1999); Laura K. Guerrero and Kory Floyd, *Nonverbal Communication in Close Relationships (LEA's Series on Personal Relationships)* 1st ed. (New York: Routledge, 2010).

16. Michele Scheinkman and Mona Fishbane, "The Vulnerability Cycle: Working with Impasses in Couple Therapy," *Family Process* 43, no. 3 (2004): 279–99, doi:10.1111/j.1545-5300.2004.00023.x. The vulnerability cycle was developed in the United States independent of, though parallel to, Halko Weiss's work on the reciprocal interaction loop in Germany.

17. Halko Weiss, "WW8 – ein Instrument (auch) für die Paartherapie: Die Analyse von Wechselwirkungen in kritischen dyadischen Beziehungssituationen" ("WW8 - An Instrument (also) for Couples Therapy: The Analysis of Interactions in Critical Dyadic Relationships"), *Familiendynamik* 32, no. 4 (October 2007): 330–45.

18. Scheinkman and Fishbane, "The Vulnerability Cycle," 281.
19. Rob Fisher, "Jumping Out of the System," in *Hakomi Mindfulness-Centered Somatic Psychotherapy*, ed. Halko Weiss, Greg Johanson, and Lorena Monda (New York: Norton, 2015), 242–51.
20. Mona Fishbane, *Loving with the Brain in Mind: Neurobiology and Couple Therapy* (New York: Norton, 2013).
21. Marion Solomon and Stan Tatkin, *Love and War in Intimate Relationships: Connection, Disconnection, and Mutual Regulation in Couple Therapy*, Norton Series on Interpersonal Neurobiology (New York and London: W. W. Norton, 2011).
22. Fishbane, *Loving with the Brain in Mind*.
23. Solomon and Tatkin, *Love and War in Intimate Relationships*.
24. Janice K. Kiecolt-Glaser and Stephanie J. Wilson, "Lovesick: How Couples' Relationships Influence Health," *Annual Review of Clinical Psychology* 13, no. 1 (2017): 421–43, https://doi.org/10.1146/annurev-clinpsy-032816-045111.
25. Solomon and Tatkin, *Love and War in Intimate Relationships*.
26. Stephen Porges, "Neuroception: A Subconscious System for Detecting Threats and Safety," *Zero to Three Journal* 24, no. 5 (May 2004): 19–24.
27. Joseph LeDoux, *The Emotional Brain: The Mysterious Underpinnings of Emotional Life* (New York: Simon & Schuster, 1996), 165.
28. Fishbane, *Loving with the Brain in Mind*.
29. Deb Dana, *The Polyvagal Theory in Therapy: Engaging the Rhythm of Regulation*, Norton Series on Interpersonal Neurobiology (New York: Norton, 2018).
30. Nancy Eichhorn, "Safety: The Preamble for Social Engagement, An interview with Stephen W. Porges, PhD," *Somatic Psychotherapy Today* (Spring 2012), 54, https://static1.squarespace.com/static/5c1d025fb27e390a78569537/t/5cce0254eb3931597f8fe2a4/1557004884326/Preamble-Social-Engagement-Interview-Porges-1.pdf.
31. www.goodreads.com/quotes/320600-we-can-not-solve-our-problems-with-the-same.
32. Weiss, "WW8 – ein Instrument (auch) für die Paartherapie..
33. Siegel, *The Developing Mind*.
34. Elizabeth Gilbert, *Eat, Pray, Love: One Woman's Search for Everything across Italy, India and Indonesia* (New York: Riverhead Books, Penguin Random House, 2006), 164.
35. Susan M. Johnson and Valerie E. Whiffen, *Attachment Processes in Couple and Family Therapy* (New York: Guilford Press, 2003).

36. Lynne Knobloch-Fedders,"The Importance of the Relationship with the Therapist," *Clinical Science Insights* 1, www.family-institute.org/sites/default/files/pdfs/csi_fedders_relationship_with_therapist.pdf; Lambert Michael and Dean Barley, "Research Summary of the Therapeutic Relationship and Psychotherapy Outcome," *Psychotherapy: Theory, Research, Practice, Training* 38, no. 4 (October 2001): 357–61, doi:10.1037/0033-3204.38.4.357.

37. Solomon and Tatkin, *Love and War in Intimate Relationships*, 5

38. Welwood, *Love and Awakening*, 227.

39. Siegel, *The Developing Mind*, 172.

40. Allan Schore, "The Neurobiology of Attachment and Early Personality Organization," *Journal of Prenatal & Perinatal Psychology & Health* 16, no. 3 (Spring 2002): 249–63.

41. Robert M. Sapolsky, *Why Zebras Don't Get Ulcers: The Acclaimed Guide to Stress, Stress-Related Diseases, and Coping* (New York: Holt, 2004).

42. Linda Graham, "Train Your Brain to Build Resilience," *Mindful* (blog), September 15, 2019, www.mindful.org/train-your-brain-to-build-resilience/.

43. Tatkin, *Wired for Love.*

44. This term was coined by Daniel Siegel in *The Mindful Brain*, 215. See also Daphne David and Jeffrey Hayes, "What Are the Benefits of Mindfulness? A Practice Review of Psychotherapy-Related Research," *Psychotherapy: Theory, Research, Practice, Training* 48, no. 2 (June 2011): 198–208, doi:10.1037/a0022062.

45. Tatkin, *Wired for Love.*

46. Linda Graham, *Bouncing Back: Rewiring Your Brain for Maximum Resilience and Well-Being* (Novato, CA: New World Library, 2013).

47. Dana, *The Polyvagal Theory in Therapy.*

48. Daniel Goleman and Richard Davidson, *Altered Traits: Science Reveals How Meditation Changes Your Mind, Brain, and Body* (New York: Penguin/Random House, 2017).

49. Heidemarie K. Laurent et al., "Mindfulness during Romantic Conflict Moderates the Impact of Negative Partner Behaviors on Cortisol Responses," *Hormones and Behavior* 79 (March 2016): 45–51, doi:10.1016/j.yhbeh.2016.01.005.

50. Jett Psaris and Marlena Lyons, *Undefended Love* (Oakland, CA: New Harbinger Publications, 2000), 18.

51. Scheinkman and Fishbane, "The Vulnerability Cycle.

52. Halko Weiss, personal communication, 2007.

53. Mindful self-study is a core skill of Hakomi Mindful Somatic Psychotherapy. See *Hakomi Mindfulness-Centered Somatic Psychotherapy,* ed. Halko Weiss, Greg Johanson, and Lorena Monda (New York: Norton, 2015).

54. Kristin Neff and Christopher Germer, "Self-Compassion and Psychological Well-Being," in *Oxford Handbook of Compassion Science,* ed. Emma M. Seppälä et al. (Oxford: Oxford University Press, 2017), 371–86.

55. Cathy W. Hall et al., "The Role of Self-Compassion in Physical and Psychological Well-Being," *The Journal of Psychology* 147, no. 4 (July–August 2013): 311–23, https://doi.org/10.1080/00223980.2012.693138.

56. Kristin Neff and S. Natasha Beretvas, "The Role of Self-Compassion in Romantic Relationships," *Self and Identity* 12, no. 1 (2012): 1–21, doi:10.108 0/15298868.2011.639548.

57. Lisa Yarnell and Kristin Neff, "Self-Compassion, Interpersonal Conflict Resolutions, and Well-Being," *Self and Identity* 12, no. 2 (2012): 146–59, doi :10.1080/15298868.2011.649545.

58. Jennifer Crocker and Katherine M. Knight, "Contingencies of Self-Worth," *Current Directions in Psychological Science* 14, no. 4 (August 2005): 200–203. doi:10.1111/j.0963-7214.2005.00364.x. See myth #4 in Kristin Neff's "The 5 Myths of Self-Compassion," *Psychotherapy Networker* (blog), September/October 2015, www.psychotherapynetworker.org/magazine /article/4/the-5-myths-of-self-compassion.

59. Kristin Neff, "Self-Compassion, Self-Esteem, and Well-Being," *Social and Personality Psychology Compass* 5, no. 1 (2011): 1–12, 10.1111/j .1751-9004.2010.00330.x; Jennifer Crocker and Lora E. Park, "The Costly Pursuit of Self-Esteem," *Psychological Bulletin* 130, no. 3 (June 2004): 392–414, https://doi.org/10.1037/0033-2909.130.3.392.

60. Brad J. Bushman et al., "Looking Again, and Harder, for a Link between Low Self-Esteem and Aggression," *Journal of Personality* 77, no. 2 (April 2009): 427–46, doi:10.1111/j.1467-6494.2008.00553.x.

61. Mayte Navarro-Gil et al., "Effects of Attachment-Based Compassion Therapy (ABCT) on Self-Compassion and Attachment Style in Healthy People," *Mindfulness* (January 2018), doi: 10.1007/ s12671-018-0896-1.

62. Christopher Germer and Sharon Salzberg, *The Mindful Path to Self-Compassion: Freeing Yourself from Destructive Thoughts and Emotions* (New York: Guilford Press, 2009).

63. Psaris and Lyons, *Undefended Love,* 21.

64. James Baldwin, *The Fire Next Time* (1962; New York: Vintage Books/Random House, 1991).

65. Welwood, *Love and Awakening*, 134.

66. Daniel Goleman, "Brain's Design Emerges as a Key to Emotions," *New York Times*, August 15, 1989, section C, 1, www.nytimes.com/1989/08/15/science/brain-s-design-emerges-as-a-key-to-emotions.html.

67. Scheinkman and Fishbane, "The Vulnerability Cycle," 291.

68. Weiss, "WW8 – ein Instrument (auch) für die Paartherapie."

69. Ed Tronick, "Typical and Atypical Development: Peek-a-boo and Blind Selection," in *Infant and Early Childhood Mental Health: Core Concepts and Clinical Practice*, ed. Kristie Brandt et al. (Washington, DC: American Psychiatric Publishing, 2014), 55–70.

70. Psaris and Lyons, *Undefended Love*, 52.

71. Fred Luskin, "Fred Luskin on Overcoming the Pain of Intimacy," *Greater Good Magazine* (blog), February 11, 2012, https://greatergood.berkeley.edu/article/item/fred_luskin_on_overcoming_the_pain_of_intimacy.

72. www.brainyquote.com/quotes/lao_tzu_101043.

## CHAPTER 4: EROTIC TRANSFORMATION

1. www.brainyquote.com/quotes/frank_a_clark_156704.

2. Edward Tronic and Bruce Perry, "Multiple Levels of Meaning-Making: The First Principles of Changing Meanings and Development in Therapy," in *The Handbook of Body Psychotherapy and Somatic Psychology*, ed. Gustl Marlock et al. (Berkeley, CA: North Atlantic Books, 2015), 345–55.

3. Inge Bretherton and Kristine A. Munholland, "Internal Working Models in Attachment Relationships: Elaborating a Central Construct in Attachment Theory," in *Handbook of Attachment: Theory, Research, and Clinical Applications*, ed. Jude Cassidy and Phillip R. Shaver (New York: The Guilford Press, 2008), 102–27.

4. Claudia G. Ucros, "Mood State-Dependent Memory: A Meta-Analysis," *Cognition and Emotion* 3, no. 2 (1989): 139–69, doi:10.1080/02699938908408077.

5. Stacey Colino, "Are You Catching Other People's Emotions?" *U.S. News* (blog), January 20, 2016, https://health.usnews.com/health-news/health-wellness/articles/2016-01-20/are-you-catching-other-peoples-emotions.

6. Cozolino, Louis J., *The Neuroscience of Relationships: Attachment and the Developing Social Brain* (New York: W. W. Norton, 2006).

7. Judith R. Schore and Allan N. Schore, "Modern Attachment Theory: The Central Role of Affect Regulation in Development and Treatment," *Clinical Social Work Journal* 36, no. 1 (September 2007), 9–20, doi:10.1007/s10615-007-0111-7.

8. Paula Pietromonaco and Lisa Barrett, "The Internal Working Models Concept: What Do We Really Know about the Self in Relation to Others?" *Review of General Psychology* 4 (2000): 155–75, doi:10.1037/1089-2680.4.2.155.

9. Siegel, *The Developing Mind*.

10. Cherry, "How Confirmation Bias Works."

11. Mauricio Cortina and Giovanni Liotti, "New Approaches to Understanding Unconscious Processes: Implicit and Explicit Memory Systems," *International Forum of Psychoanalysis* 16, no. 4 (2007): 204–12, doi:10.1080/08037060701676326.

12. Sharon Begley, *Train Your Mind, Change Your Brain* (New York: Ballantine Books, 2007), 61.

13. Efrat Ginot, "A Neuropsychological Model of the Unconscious and Therapeutic Change," *Science of Psychology* (blog), July 2, 2015, www.thescienceofpsychotherapy.com/a-neuropsychological-model-of-the-unconscious-and-therapeutic-change/.

14. Mark Spiering, Walter Everaerd, and Erick Janseen, "Priming the Sexual System: Implicit versus Explicit Activation," *The Journal of Sex Research* 40, no. 2 (May 2003): 134–45.

15. Esther Heerema, "How Does Dementia Affect Long-Term Memory? Long-Term Memory Loss in Alzheimer's," *Verywellhealth* (blog), June 24, 2019, www.verywellhealth.com/long-term-memory-and-alzheimers-98562.

16. Marilyn Morgan, "The Body Unconscious: The Process of Making Conscious: Psychodynamic and Neuroscience Perspectives," in *The Handbook of Body Psychotherapy and Somatic Psychology*, ed. Gustl Marlock et al. (Berkeley, CA: North Atlantic Books, 2015), 219–29.

17. Bessel van der Kolk, *The Body Keeps the Score: Brain, Mind, and Body in the Healing of Trauma* (New York: Penguin Books, 2015), 44.

18. Christine Caldwell, "Sensation, Movement, and Emotion: Explicit Procedures for Implicit Memories," in *Body Memory, Metaphor and Movement, Advances in Consciousness Research*, 84, ed. Sabine C. Koch et al. (Amsterdam: John Benjamins Publishing Company, 2012), 255–65.

19. Siegel, *The Developing Mind*, 46.

20. Siegel, *The Developing Mind*, 48.

21. Personal communication with Cedar Barstow, 2018, who coined the term in a therapy session. Barstow used the word in a different context but gave me permission to apply my definition to stage 3 coupling.

22. Ron Kurtz, "Bodily Expression and Experience in Body Psychotherapy," in *The Handbook of Body Psychotherapy and Somatic Psychology*, ed. Gustl Marlock et al. (Berkeley, CA: North Atlantic Books, 2015), 411–18.

23. Eugene Gendlin and Marion N. Hendricks-Gendlin, "The Bodily 'Felt Sense' as a Ground for Body Psychotherapies," in *The Handbook of Body Psychotherapy and Somatic Psychology*, ed. Gustl Marlock et al. (Berkeley, CA: North Atlantic Books, 2015), 248–54.

24. Halko Weiss and Maci Daye, "The Art of Bottom-Up Processing: Mindfulness, Meaning, and Self-Compassion in Body-Psychotherapy," in *The Routledge International Handbook of Embodied Perspectives in Psychotherapy: Approaches from Dance Movement and Body Psychotherapies*, ed. Helen Payne et al. (New York: Routledge International Handbooks, 2019), 273–82.

25. Christian Gottwald, "Neurobiological Perspectives in Body Psychotherapy," in *Hakomi Mindfulness-Centered Somatic Psychotherapy*, ed. Halko Weiss, Greg Johanson, and Lorena Monda (New York: Norton, 2015), 126–47.

26. Jellaludin Rumi, "There's Nothing Ahead," *Rumi: The Book of Love Poems of Ecstasy and Longing*, trans. Coleman Barks (New York: HarperCollins, 2003), 205.

27. Schnarch, *Passionate Marriage*, 66.

28. Couple's therapists may wish to consult Rob Fisher's book, *Experiential Psychotherapy with Couples: A Guide for the Creative Pragmatist* (Phoenix, AZ: Zeig Tucker & Theisen, 2002), to source other experiential techniques.

29. Brach, Tara, *Radical Acceptance: Embracing Your Life With the Heart of a Buddha* (New York: Bantam, 2004), 52.

30. Weiss and Daye, "The Art of Bottom-Up Processing."

31. Brené Brown, *The Gifts of Imperfection: Let Go of Who You Think You're Supposed to Be And Embrace Who You Are* (Center City, Minnesota: Hazelton, 2010).

32. Maci Daye, "The Experimental Attitude: Curiosity in Action," in *Hakomi Mindfulness-Centered Somatic Psychotherapy*, ed. Halko Weiss, Greg Johanson, and Lorena Monda (New York: Norton, 2015), 120–28; Richard D. Lane et al., "Memory Reconsolidation, Emotional Arousal, and the Process of Change in Psychotherapy: New Insights from Brain Science," *Behavioral and Brain Sciences* 38 (2015), E1, doi:10.1017/S0140525X14000041; Karim Nader, "Memory Traces Unbound," *Trends in Neurosciences* 26, no. 2 (2003), 65–72.

33. Bruce Ecker, "Understanding Memory Reconsolidation," *The Neuropsychotherapist* (January 2015): 4–22, doi:10.12744/tnpt(10)004-022.

34. Carl Jung, "The Philosophical Tree," in *Collected Works 13: Alchemical Studies* (Princeton, NJ: Princeton University Press, 1967), paragraph 335.

35. Peter A. Levine and Ann Frederick, *Waking the Tiger: Healing Trauma* (Berkeley, CA: North Atlantic Books, 1997).

36. I recommend you locate a Somatic Experiencing or Sensorimotor practitioner. Here are the practitioner directories at both organizations: https://directory.traumahealing.org/?gml=400 and www.sensorimotorpsycho therapy.org/directory.html.

37. Emily Nagoski, "The Truth about Unwanted Arousal," TED talk, June 4, 2018, 15:17 www.youtube.com/watch?v=L-q-tSH09H0&list=PLT5KTlgIixI XMRTs5PHJsjDhYlLok3J2s; Kelly D. Suschinsky and Martin L. Lalumière, "Prepared for Anything? An Investigation of Female Genital Arousal in Response to Rape Cues," *Psychological Science* 22, no. 2 (2010): 159–65, doi:10.1177/0956797610394660.

38. The notion of completing a truncated fight response is central to the idea of "renegotiating" a trauma in Somatic Experiencing.

39. These techniques come from Somatic Experiencing, a somatic trauma theory developed by Peter Levine; see his *Waking the Tiger.*

40. Courtney E. Ackerman, "What Is Neuroplasticity? A Psychologist Explains [+14 Exercises]," *PositivePsychology.com* (blog), September 10, 2019, https://positivepsychology.com/neuroplasticity/.

41. Schwartz and Begley, *The Mind and the Brain.*

42. For more on this subject, see thebodyisnotanapology.com/magazine/sex-with-the-non-binary-person-even-when-that-person-is-you-maya/

## CHAPTER 5: EROTIC EXPRESSION

1. Joy Davidson, *Fearless Sex: A Babe's Guide to Overcoming Your Romantic Obsessions and Getting the Sex Life You Deserve* (Gloucester, MA: Fair Winds Press, 2004), 33.

2. Shawn Levy, *Date Night,* Directed by Shawn Levy, 20th Century Fox, Los Angeles, CA, 2010.

3. Anaïs Nin, *Henry and June: From a Journal of Love—The Unexpurgated Diary of Anaïs Nin, 1931–1932* (San Diego, CA: Harcourt, 1989), 2.

4. Davidson, *Fearless Sex,* 33.

5. David Schnarch, *Intimacy & Desire: Awaken the Passion in Your Relationship* (New York: Beaufort Books, 2009); Richard Schwartz, "Pathways to Sexual Intimacy: Revealing Our Many Selves in the Bedroom," *Psychotherapy Networker* (blog), May/June 2003, originally published as "Rediscovering Pleasure: Are Therapists Afraid of Eroticism?" *Psychotherapy Networker,* 27, no. 3.

6. www.goodreads.com/quotes/348178-shame-is-the-lie-someone-told-you-about-yourself.

7. Ana Fortes and Vinícius Ferreira, "The Influence of Shame in Social Behavior," *Revista de Psicologia da IMED* 6 no. 1 (January–June 2014): 25–27, doi:10.18256/2175-5027/psico-imed.v6n1; Joseph Burgo, "Shame Is Known as a Toxic Feeling. But It Can Also Be a Force for Good," *Vox* (blog), April 18, 2019, ww.vox.com/first-person/2019/4/18/18308346/shame-toxic-productive.

8. Brené Brown, *Daring Greatly: How the Courage to Be Vulnerable Transforms the Way We Live, Love, Parent, and Lead* (New York: Avery/Penguin Random House, 2012), 69.

9. Ida Strøm et al., "The Mediating Role of Shame in the Relationship between Childhood Bullying Victimization and Adult Psychosocial Adjustment," *European Journal of Psychotraumatology* 9, no. 1, (2018): 1–13, doi:10.1080/20008198.2017.1418570.

10. Annette Kämmerer, "The Scientific Underpinnings and Impacts of Shame," *Scientific American* (blog), August 9, 2019, www.scientificamerican.com/author/annette-kaemmerer/.

11. Noel Clark, "The Etiology and Phenomenology of Sexual Shame: A Grounded Theory Study," *Clinical Psychology Dissertations*, 25 (2017): 87, https://digitalcommons.spu.edu/cpy_etd/25.

12. *Merriam-Webster's Dictionary*, www.merriam-webster.com/dictionary/pudendum.

13. Douglas Jehl, "Surgeon General Forced to Resign by White House," *New York Times*, December 10, 1994, www.nytimes.com/1994/12/10/us/surgeon-general-forced-to-resign-by-white-house.html.

14. Dan Evon, "Is It Illegal to Have More Than Two Dildos in a Home in Arizona?" *Snopes.com* (blog), February 6, 2019, www.snopes.com/fact-check/arizona-dildo-law/; Sarah Boboltz, "8 Laws to Keep Women in Line That Are Somehow Still on the Books," *HuffPost* (blog), March 14, 2014, www.huffpost.com/entry/state-laws-women_n_4937387; D. Savage, *Savage Love*.

15. Suzanne Iasenza, "What Is Queer About Sex? Expanding Sexual Frames in Theory and Practice," *Family Process* 49, no. 3 (2010): 291–308.

16. Robert Sapolsky, *Behave: The Biology of Humans at Our Best and Worst* (New York: Penguin Books, 2018).

17. Ann Haas, Philip Rodgers, and Jody Herman, *Suicide Attempts among Transgender and Gender Non-Conforming Adults, Findings of the National Transgender Discrimination Survey* (American Foundation for Suicide Prevention, The Williams Institute, 2014).

18. Davidson, *Fearless Sex*, 65.

19. Psaris and Lyons, *Undefended Love*, 101.
20. www.goodreads.com/quotes/99661-the-truly-faithless-one-is-the-one-who-makes-love.
21. Tammy Nelson, *When You're The One Who Cheats: Ten Things You Need to Know* (Toronto: RL Publishing Corp, 2019).
22. Schwartz, "Pathways to Sexual Intimacy."
23. Richard Schwartz, *Internal Family Systems* (New York: Guilford, 1995).
24. Nin, *Henry and June*, 83.
25. Personal communication, December 11, 2019. Terrence Real is the founder of the Relational Life Institute, at www.terryreal.com.
26. Esther Perel, *Mating in Captivity: Reconciling the Erotic and the Domestic* (New York: Harper Collins, 2006), 217.
27. Rose Eveleth, "Americans Are More into BDSM Than the Rest of the World," *Smithsonian.com*, February 10, 2014, www.smithsonianmag.com /smart-news/americans-are-more-bdsm-rest-world-180949703/.
28. E. L. James, *Fifty Shades of Grey* (New York: Vintage Books/Random House, 2012).
29. Welwood, *Journey of the Heart*, 180.
30. Rasheta, "The Three Poisons."
31. David Schnarch, "Sexual Relationships Always Consist of 'Leftovers'," *Psychology Today*, June 1, 2011 (blog), www.psychologytoday.com/intl/blog /intimacy-and-desire/201106/sexual-relationships-always-consist-leftovers.
32. Davidson, *Fearless Sex*, 118–19.
33. Jack Morin, *The Erotic Mind: Unlocking the Inner Sources of Sexual Passion and Fulfillment* (New York: Harper Collins, 1996).
34. Schwartz, "Pathways to Sexual Intimacy"; "Richard Schwartz on Better Sex through the IFS Approach," *Psychotherapy Networker* (blog), February 3, 2015, www.psychotherapynetworker.org/blog/details/508/internal-family-systems-guidepost-for-sexual-intimacy; Maci Daye and Richard Schwartz, *Bringing More of Ourselves to the Bedroom*, June 27, 2019, www .youtube.com/watch?v=kGqSLinBqyc&feature=youtu.be.
35. Schwartz, "Pathways to Sexual Intimacy"; "Richard Schwartz on Better Sex through the IFS Approach"; Daye and Schwartz, *Bringing More of Ourselves to the Bedroom*.
36. Schwartz, "Pathways to Sexual Intimacy"; "Richard Schwartz on Better Sex through the IFS Approach"; Daye and Schwartz, *Bringing More of Ourselves to the Bedroom*.
37. Suggested resources for having these conversations are Mark Michaels and Patricia Johnson, *Partners in Passion: A Guide to Great Sex, Emotional*

*Intimacy, and Long-Term Love* (Berkeley, CA: Cleis Press, 2014), and Tammy Nelson, *The New Monogamy: Redefining Your Relationship after Infidelity.* (Oakland, CA: New Harbinger Publications, 2013).

38. Ian Kerner, *Passionista: The Empowered Woman's Guide to Pleasuring a Man* (William Morrow Paperbacks, 2008), 83.

39. Michael Ventura, "Journey to the In-Between," *Psychotherapy Networker* (blog), November-December 2009, www.psychotherapynetworker.org /magazine/article/468/journey-to-the-in-between.

40. Nespresso VertuoLine. "The Quest." Television advertisement. Untitled Inc, directed by Grant Heslov, 2018.

41. Peter Gabriel, "Solsbury Hill," *Peter Gabriel,* 1977, Atco Records/Charisma Records, vinyl record.

## CHAPTER 6: EROTIC ATTUNEMENT

1. Lao-Tzu, chapter 23, in *Tao Te Ching,* trans. Stephen Mitchell (New York: HarperPerennial, 1988).

2. Morin, *The Erotic Mind.*

3. Peggy Kleinplatz, *Extraordinary Erotic Intimacy: Lessons for Lovers and Sex Therapists: The Sexual Reawakening Summit, Love, Intimacy, Sexual Desire,* hosted by Dr. Erica Goodstone, 2016, https://sexualreawakening.org/peggy/.

4. "Contact improvisation is an evolving system of movement initiated in 1972 by American choreographer Steve Paxton. The improvised dance form is based on the communication between two moving bodies that are in physical contact and their combined relationship to the physical laws that govern their motion—gravity, momentum, inertia. The body, in order to open to these sensations, learns to release excess muscular tension and abandon a certain quality of willfulness to experience the natural flow of movement." See https://contactquarterly.com/contact-improvisation /about/. See also www.contactimprov.com/whatiscontactimprov.html.

5. Eugene Gendlin, *Focusing* (1978; New York: Bantam Books/Random House, 2007).

6. Benny Golson, https://lindagraham-mft.net/weekly-quotes-2014/.

7. Kahlil Gibran, "On Children," in *The Prophet* (New York: Knopf, 1994), 17.

8. The 10,000-hour figure was cited in Malcolm Gladwell's book *Outliers.* However, the following resources explain that time alone does not lead to mastery: Shana Lebowitz, "A Top Psychologist Says There's Only One Way to Become the Best in Your Field—But Not Everyone Agrees," *Business Insider Deutschland* (blog), February 2, 2018, www.businessinsider.de/anders-ericsson-how-to-become-an-expert-at-anything-2016-6?r=US&IR=T.

9. Brooke N. Macnamara, David Moreau, and David Z. Hambrick, "The Relationship between Deliberate Practice and Performance in Sports: A Meta-Analysis," *Perspectives on Psychological Science* 11, no. 3, (2016): 333–50, https://doi.org/10.1177/1745691616635591.

10. Welwood, *Journey of the Heart*, 181.

11. John H. Holland, *Hidden Order: How Adaptation Builds Complexity* (New York: Perseus Books Group, 1995).

12. Alan Alda, commencement speech at Connecticut College, 1980, www .graduationwisdom.com/speeches/0020-alda1.htm.

13. Daniel Siegel, *The Mindful Therapist: A Clinician's Guide to Mindsight and Neural Integration* (New York: W. W. Norton, 2010), 10, figure 1.1.

14. Siegel, *Aware*.

15. Sara W. Lazar et al., "Meditation Experience Is Associated with Increased Cortical Thickness," *Neuroreport* 16, no. 17 (2005): 1893–97, doi:10.1097/01 .wnr.0000186598.66243.19.

16. Welwood, *Journey of the Heart*, 175.

17. Ellen Langer, Timothy Russel, and Noah Eisenkraft, "Orchestral Performance and the Footprint of Mindfulness," *Psychology of Music* 37, no. 2 (2009): 125–36, https://doi.org/10.1177/0305735607086053.

18. George Lois, *Damn Good Advice (for People with Talent!): How to Unleash Your Creative Potential by America's Master Communicator* (New York: Phaidon, 2012), 10.

19. https://quotepark.com/authors/henri-frederic-amiel/.

20. Gordon Kerry, "The Impermanence of Being: Toward a Psychology Of Uncertainty," *Journal of Humanistic Psychology* 43 (2003): 96–117, doi:10.1177/0022167802250731, 107.

21. Welwood, *Journey of the Heart*, 181.

22. Keith Sawyer and Stacy Dezutter, "Distributed Creativity: How Collective Creations Emerge from Collaboration," *Psychology of Aesthetics, Creativity, and the Arts* 3, no. 2 (2009): 81–92, doi:10.1037/a0013282.

23. Julie Daley, "Embodiment: Lighting the Temple from Within," *Unabashedlyfemale* (blog), November 24, 2009, www.unabashedlyfemale .com/2009/11/24/embodiment-lighting-the-temple-from-within/.

24. For more ideas on becoming embodied, see Alan Fogel, *Body Sense: The Science and Practice of Embodied Self-Awareness*, Norton Series on Interpersonal Neurobiology, 1st ed. (New York: W. W. Norton, 2009).

25. Martha Lee, "6 Ways to Be Mindfully Zen During Sex for SERIOUSLY Intense Orgasms," *YourTango* (blog), June 27, 2016, www.yourtango.com /experts/dr-martha-lee/how-practice-mindfulness-during-sex.

26. Brown, *The Gifts of Imperfection*.
27. www.brainyquote.com/quotes/albert_einstein_148788.
28. Marty Klein, *Sexual Intelligence: What We Really Want from Sex—and How to Get It* (New York: Harper Collins, 2012), 20.
29. Edward Tronick and Marjorie Beeghly, "Infants' Meaning-Making and the Development of Mental Health Problems," *American Psychology* 66, no. 2 (2011): 107–19, doi:10.1037/a0021631, 114.
30. Michael Freeman, "There's a New Sex Toy for Men, and It's Called 'The Guybrator' (NSFW)," *thejournal.ie* (blog), August 24, 2015, https://jrnl.ie/2289868.

## CHAPTER 7: EROTIC SUSTENANCE

1. Tom Robbins, *Still Life with Woodpecker: A Novel* (New York: Bantam Books/ Random House, 2003), 151.
2. Klein, *Sexual Intelligence*, 25.
3. Leonore Tiefer, "In Pursuit of the Perfect Penis: The Medicalization of Male Sexuality," *American Behavioral Scientist* 29, no. 5 (May/June 1986), 579–99, https://doi.org/10.1177/000276486029005006.
4. A. H. Almaas, *Elements of the Real in Man* (Boulder, CO: Shambhala, 1987), 128.
5. Schnarch, *Passionate Marriage*.
6. Michael Metz and Barry McCarthy, *Enduring Desire: Your Guide to Lifelong Intimacy* (New York and London: Routledge, 2011), 18.
7. Melissa Conrad Stöppler, "The Surprising Health Benefits of Sex," *On-Health.com* (blog), April 2, 2016, www.onhealth.com/content/1/health_benefits_sex.
8. Anthony Smith et al., "Sexual and Relationship Satisfaction among Heterosexual Men and Women: The Importance of Desired Frequency of Sex," *Sex Marital Therapy* 37, no. 2 (2011): 104–15, doi:10.1080/00926 23X.2011.560531.
9. Julia Heiman et al., "Sexual Satisfaction and Relationship Happiness in Midlife and Older Couples in Five Countries," *Archives of Sexual Behavior* 40 (2011): 741–53, doi:10.1007/s10508-010-9703-3.
10. Jen Gunter, "Treating the Incredible Shrinking Vagina: What Is 'Vaginal Atrophy,' and How Can You Stop It?" *New York Times* (blog), September 19, 2019, https://nyti.ms/2SO8HQP.
11. Suzy Strutner, "Sitting All Day Is Even More Dangerous Than We Thought," *Huffpost* (blog), updated September 14, 2017, www.huffpost.com/entry/sitting-health-effects_n_57b4b4e3e4b095b2f5421a58.

12. Yuri Hanin, "Emotions and Athletic Performance: Individual Zones of Optimal Functioning Model," *European Yearbook of Sport Psychology* 1 (1997): 29–72.

13. Pat Ogden, Kekuni Minton, and Clare Pain, *Trauma and the Body: A Sensorimotor Approach to Psychotherapy* (New York: Norton, 2006); Siegel, *The Developing Mind.*

14. Amelia M. Stanton, Ariel B. Handy, and Cindy M. Meston, "The Effects of Exercise on Sexual Function in Women," *Sexual Medicine Reviews* 6, no. 4 (October 2018): 548–57, https://doi.org/10.1016/j.sxmr.2018.02.004; Cindy Meston and Amelia Stanton, "Exercise and Sexual Arousal in Women: The Effects of Acute Exercise on Physiological Sexual Arousal in Women," *The Sexual Psychopysiology Laboratory*, https://labs.la.utexas.edu/meston-lab/?page_id=1434.

15. Tierney Ahrold Lorenz et al., "Evidence for a Curvilinear Relationship between Sympathetic Nervous System Activation and Women's Physiological Sexual Arousal," *Psychophysiology* 49, no. 1 (January 2012): 111–17, doi:10.1111/j.1469-8986.2011.01285.x.

16. Tierney Ahrold Lorenz and Cindy M. Meston, "Exercise Improves Sexual Function in Women Taking Antidepressants: Results from a Randomized Crossover Trial," *Depression and Anxiety* 31, no. 3, (2014): 188–95, doi:10.1002/da.22208.

17. Cindy M. Meston and Boris B. Gorzalka, "Differential Effects of Sympathetic Activation on Sexual Arousal in Sexually Dysfunctional and Functional Women," *Journal of Abnormal Psychology* 105, no. 4, (1996): 582–91, https://doi.org/10.1037/0021-843X.105.4.582.

18. John Clarke, "Soothe Your Nervous System with 2-1 Breathing," *YogaInternational* (blog), https://yogainternational.com/article/view/soothe-your-nervous-system-with-2-to-1-breathing.

19. Vikas Dhikav et al., "Yoga in Female Sexual Functions," *The Journal of Sexual Medicine* 7, no. 2 (February 2010): 964–70, doi:10.1111/j.1743-6109.2009.01580.x.

20. Edward McAuley, Shannon Mihalko, and Susan Bane, "Exercise and Self-Esteem in Middle-Aged Adults: Multidimentional Relationships and Physical Fitness and Self-Efficacy Influences," *Journal of Behavioral Medicine* 20, no. 1 (1997): 67–83.

21. Angela Weaver and Sandra Byers, "The Relationships among Body Image, Body Mass Index, Exercise, and Sexual Functioning in Heterosexual Women," *Psychology of Women Quarterly* 30 (2006): 333–39

22. Amanda Ravary, Mark W. Baldwin, Jennifer A. Bartz, "Shaping the Body Politic: Mass Media Fat-Shaming Affects Implicit Anti-Fat Attitudes," *Personality and Social Psychology Bulletin* 45 (April 2019), doi:10.1177/0146167219838550; "Celebrity Fat Shaming has Ripple Effects on Women's Implicit Anti-Fat Attitudes," *ScienceDaily, Society for Personality and Social Psychology*, April 15, 2019, www.sciencedaily.com /releases/2019/04/190415082001.htm; Michael Wiederman, "Women's Body Image Self-Consciousness during Physical Intimacy with a Partner," *Journal of Sex Research* 37, no. 1 (2000): 60–68, doi:10.1080/00224490009552021.

23. Klein, *Sexual Intelligence*, 186.

24. Schnarch, *Passionate Marriage*, 76.

25. Schnarch, *Passionate Marriage*, 78.

26. If you are struggling with sexual side effects from prostate cancer, I highly recommend this resource: Jeffrey Albaugh, *Reclaiming Sex and Intimacy after Prostate Cancer* (Sewell, NY: Jannetti Publications 2018).

27. Barry McCarthy and Lana Wald, "Mindfulness and Good Enough Sex," *Sexual & Relationship Therapy* 28 (2013), https://doi.org/10.1080/14681994 .2013.770829.

28. Kerner, *Passionista*, 86. See also, Ian Kerner, *She Comes First: The Thinking Man's Guide to Pleasuring a Woman* (New York: William Morrow Paperbacks, 2010).

29. Klein, *Sexual Intelligence*, 141.

30. Michael Mertz and Barry McCarthy, "The Good Enough Sex Model for Couple Sexual Satisfaction," *Sexual and Relationship Therapy* 22, no. 3 (2007): 351–62, doi:10.1080/14681990601013492.

31. E. Sandra Byers, "Relationship Satisfaction and Sexual Satisfaction: A Longitudinal Study of Individuals in Long-Term Relationships," *The Journal of Sex Research* 42, no. 2 (May 2005): 113–18, www.jstor.org /stable/3813147.

32. Cheryl Fraser, *Buddha's Bedroom: The Mindful Loving Path to Sexual Passion and Lifelong Intimacy* (Oakland, CA: Reveal Press, 2019), 1.

33. Suzanne Iasenza, "Transforming Sexual Narratives: From Dysfunction to Discovery," *PsychotherapyNetworker.org* (blog), January–February 2016, 25–45, www.psychotherapynetworker.org/magazine/article/994/ transforming-sexual-narratives.

34. Rosemary Basson, "The Female Sexual Response: A Different Model," *Journal of Sex & Marital Therapy* 26, no. 1 (2000): 51–65, doi:10.1080/009262300278641.

35. Emily Nagoski, *Come as You Are: The Surprising New Science That Will Transform Your Sex Life* (New York: Simon and Shuster, 2015). Nagoski based her book on the dual-control model of arousal originally developed by researchers of the Kinsey Institute, see Erick Janssen and John Bancroft, "The Dual-Control Model: The Role of Sexual Inhibition and Excitation in Sexual Arousal and Behavior," in the Kinsey Institute Series, The Psychophysiology of Sex, ed. Janssen (Bloomington, IN: Indiana University Press, 2007), 197–222.

36. C. Sue Carter, "The Oxytocin-Vasopressin Pathway in the Context of Love and Fear," *Frontiers in Endocrinology* 8 (December 2017): 356, doi:10.3389/fendo.2017.00356.

37. Stephen Porges, *A Neural Love Code: The Body's Need to Engage and Bond*, April 19, 2013, DVD.

38. Kerstin Uvnäs-Moberg, *The Oxytocin Factor: Tapping The Hormone of Calm, Love, and Healing*, trans. Roberta Francis (Cambridge, MA: Da Capo Press, 2003).

39. Kahlil Gibran, "On Marriage," in *The Prophet*, 15–16.

40. Sue Johnson, "Episode 82: How Safety Leads to Better Sex—Sue Johnson," Relationship Alive, YouTube video, 0:58, March 15, 2017, www.youtube.com/watch?v=o7hbN2A1wgU.

41. Morin, *The Erotic Mind*.

42. Perel, *Mating in Captivity*, xv.

43. Bianca P. Acevedo et al., "Neural Correlates of Long-Term Intense Romantic Love," *Social Cognition and Affective Neuroscience* 7, no. 2 (2012): 145–59; doi:10.1093/scan/nsq092.

44. Chelom E. Leavitt, Eva S. Lefkowitz, and Emily A. Waterman, "The Role of Sexual Mindfulness in Sexual Wellbeing, Relational Wellbeing, and Self-Esteem," *Journal of Sex and Marital Therapy* 45, no. 6 (2019): 497–509, doi:10.1080/0092623X.2019.1572680.

45. Anna Kozlowski, "Mindful Mating: Exploring the Connection between Mindfulness and Relationship Satisfaction," *Sexual and Relationship Therapy* 28, nos. 1–2 (February 2013): 92–104, doi:10.1080/14681994.2012.748889; James Carson, Kimberly Carson, and Karen M. Gil, "Mindfulness-Based Relationship Enhancement," *Behavior Therapy* 35 (2004): 471–94, doi:10.1016/S0005-7894(04)80028-5.

46. Welwood, *Love and Awakening*, 6.

47. Gesa Kappen et al., "On the Association between Mindfulness and Romantic Relationship Satisfaction: The Role of Partner Acceptance," *Mindfulness* 9, no. 5 (2018): 1543–56, doi:10.1007/s12671-018-0902-7.

48. Sean Barnes et al., "The Role of Mindfulness in Romantic Relationship Satisfaction and Responses to Relationship Stress," *Journal of Marital and Family Therapy* 33, no. 4 (October 2007): 482–500.

49. Laurent et al., "Mindfulness during Romantic Conflict Moderates the Impact of Negative Partner Behaviors on Cortisol Responses."

50. Leslie C. Burpee and Ellen J. Langer, "Mindfulness and Marital Satisfaction," *Journal of Adult Development* 12 (2005): 43–51, doi:10.1007/s10804-005-1281-6.

51. Suchitra Roy Chowdhury, "Impact of Mindfulness on Anxiety and Well-Being," *Journal of Psychosocial Research*, July–December 2017, www.questia.com/library/journal/1P4-2015379615/impact-of-mindfulness-on-anxiety-and-well-being.

52. Asimina Lazaridou and Christina Kalogianni, "Mindfulness and Sexuality," *Sexual and Relationship Therapy* 28, nos. 1–2 (2013): 29–38, https://doi.org/10.1080/14681994.2013.773398.

53. Albert Einstein, "The World As I See It," *Ideas and Opinions, based on Mein Weltbild*, ed. Carl Seelig (New York: Bonzana Books, 1954), 8–11.

54. Michael Pollan, *How to Change Your Mind: The New Science of Psychedelics* (New York: Penguin Press, 2018).

55. For further information about predictive coding in perception and cognition, refer to www.quantamagazine.org/to-make-sense-of-the-present-brains-may-predict-the-future-20180710.

56. Pollan, *How to Change Your Mind*, 311.

57. Matt Killingsworth, "Does Mind-Wandering Make You Unhappy?" *Mindful* (blog), August 1, 2013, https://www.mindful.org/does-mind-wandering-make-you-unhappy/.

58. Siegel, *Aware*.

59. Moriah E. Thomason et al., "Default-Mode Function and Task-Induced Deactivation Have Overlapping Brain Substrates in Children," *Neuroimage* 41, no. 4 (July 2008): 1493–1503, doi: 10.1016/j.neuroimage.2008.03.029.

60. Kathleen A. Garrison et al., "Meditation Leads to Reduced Default Mode Network Activity beyond an Active Task," *Cognitive, Affective & Behavioral Neuroscience* 15, no. 3, (2015): 712–20, doi:10.3758/s13415-015-0358-3.

61. Judson A. Brewer et al., "Meditation Experience Is Associated with Differences in Default Mode Network Activity and Connectivity," *Proceedings of the National Academy of Sciences of the United States of America* 108, no. 50 (2011): 20254–59, doi:10.1073/pnas.1112029108.

62. Gina Ogden, *The Heart and Soul of Sex* (Boston, MA: Trumpeter, 2012), 9.

63. Ventura, "Journey to the In-Between."

64. Diane Ackerman, *A Natural History of the Senses* (New York: Penguin Random House, 1990), 309.

## ACKNOWLEDGMENTS

1. Stephanie Coontz, "Do You Take This Man? No Thanks," *Guardian*, December 30, 2006, www.theguardian.com/commentisfree/2006/dec/31/comment.gender.

# Index

*Page numbers in italics indicate figures.*

abstinence
  in stage 2 relationships, 1, 2,
    12, 185
  in stage 3 relationships, 191,
    194–95, 196
achievement mentality. *See*
  performance trance
Ackerman, Diane, 215
affairs, 23–24, 35, 36, 37, 131, 137, 141,
  153. *See also* non-monogamy
aging, 61, 185–87, 198
  physical changes from, 24,
    106–107, 189–91, 195–201
Alda, Alan, 167
Almaas, A. H., 191
Amiel, Henri Frédéric, 171
anal play, 17, 133, 187, 201, 205
animal energy, *141*, 141–42, 149, 186
anonymous sex, 141
antidepressants, 197
anxiety, 80, 143, 159, 171, 196–97
  about performance, 13, 38, 51,
    95–96, 107, 185, 200
arousal, 47–48, 76, 162, 199–201, 207
  abstinence and, 196

exercise and, 197
fantasy and, 148
illness and, 198
imprints and, 100
taking responsibility for, 202
timing of, 204
unwanted touch and, 117
attachment theory, 73, 80
attunement, 85. *See also* erotic
  attunement
automaticity, 26, 27, 33–38, 40, 41, *165*,
  166, 183
  overcoming, 37–38, 41–42, 53–60
  *See also* stage 2 relationships: as
    routine
aversion, 9, 145–46, 158, 202, 206, *211*
awakened intimacy, 6, 9–32, 217, 223
  developing, 14–16, 20–24
  exercises on, 30–32
  lack of, 9–14, 16–19, 21–30

Baldwin, James, 82
Barstow, Cedar, 218, 236*n*21
BDSM, 143
befriend cycle, 104, *105*, 107

Begley, Sharon, 99
Beretvas, Natasha, 80
biochemistry
  of aging, 189, 190, 197, 199
  of bonding, 13, *141*, 142
  of conflict, 77, 212
  of infatuation, 11, 17, 33
  of sex, 18, 141, *141*, 194, 207
birth control, 200, 207
black light syndrome, 97, 101–102,
  110, 125, 194, 223
blame, 19, 64, *104*
  avoiding, 110, 137, 202, 206, 211
  self-awareness vs., 26, 62, 65,
  74, 182
body-centered psychotherapy, 4,
  5, 164, 177, 218, 219, 238*n*36,
  238*n*38–39
body image, 51, 197–98
body scanning, 117, 175, 177
bondage, 52, 143
borrowed functioning, 107
both/and approach, 5, 223
  heart and loins, 208
  joys and challenges, 22, 43,
  44–45
  partner and self, 169–71
  pleasure and healing, 5–6, 102
  present and past, 85–86
  sinner and saint, 130
bottom-up processing, 102
Brach, Tara, 108, 164
breastfeeding, 194, 207
breasts, shame about, 113, 150
breath, 41, 121, 197
Brown, Brené, 132, 179
*Buddha's Bedroom*, 203
Buddhism, 5, 37, 38, 40,
  49, 145

Camaroto, Maryann, 29–30
cancer, 1, 194, 196, 198, 199, 245*n*26
care cycle, 81–89, *83*, 223
Carter, Sue, 207
case studies, 6
  Abbey & Quinn, 4, 5, 17–18, 19, 26
  Bella & Ezra, 181–82
  Carla & Miguel, 33–34, 35, 36, 130–
  31, 139, 148, 149–51, 152, 153, 177
  Eric & Max, 66–67, 69–70, 70–72,
  79, 82, 86–89, 99, 102, 109, 151
  Gina & Elizabeth, 54–55
  Jay & Nina, 152
  Jerome & Keisha, 4, 5, 111–12, 114,
  179–80
  Judith & Frank, 182
  Kyle & Sienna, 95–96, 101,
  103–107, 109
  Luli, 179, 180
  Mark & Stacey, 151, 152–53
  Maurice & Angela, 199, 201
  Owen & Seth, 161, 171–73
  Pam & Stuart, 1
  Riya & Nalini, 4, 5
  Sam & Wren, 124–25
  Samantha, 142
  Sara & Jerry, 185–87
  Shay & Leif, 194–95, 196
  Sue & Barney, 116–24, 219
  Walter & Ingrid, 2–3, 28, 38–39,
  51–53
childhood
  emotions from (*see* legacy states)
  sexual abuse during (*see* trauma)
  subconscious learning from (*see*
  imprint portfolios)
Chödrön, Pema, 49
chronic illness, 198–99
Clark, Frank, 95

Clark, Noel, 133
Clinton, Bill, 133
*Come as You Are*, 207
compassion, 65, 74, 80–81
compassionate contact, 84, 223
conflict, 61–74
    impasses in, 65–72, 151–53
    neuroscience of, 68–70, 77, 212
    working through, 74–94, 211–12
connected longing, 208–9
consciousness, expansion of, 141,
    212–15. *See also* mindfulness;
    perception
consent, 113, 121, 145–46, 194, 204–6
    fantasy and, 148–49, 152, 159
    somatic, 177
contact improvisation, 162, 241n4
control, need for, 52, 78, 80, 119–21,
    148, 174
core beliefs, 98–99
couples therapy, 67. *See also* case
    studies
covenants, relational, 201–202
creativity. *See* erotic attunement;
    goal-free sex; parts play; pure
    erotic potential
cultural messages
    about body image, 198
    about emotions, 22
    about kink, 143
    about mindfulness, 41
    about perfectionism, 38, 50, 165
    about "real" sex, 115–16, 190,
    200–201
    about romance, 21, 28, 73, 84–85
    about sexiness, 50, 98, 139
    sex-negative, 6, 29, 97, 133
    about shame, 132, 139
    traumatic, 78

curiosity. *See* seeing fresh
cyber sex, 153

Daley, Julie, 177
Dana, Deb, 69, 77
dancing, 152, 162, 172, 177, 184
*Date Night*, 129
dates, 203–5, 215, 216
Davidson, Joy, 129, 130, 135, 147
Davidson, Richard, 77
death, 209
default mode network, 213–14
defend cycle, 103, *104*, 109, 135
demon dialogues. *See* reciprocal
    interaction loops
dirty talk, 14
disenchantment. *See* stage 2
    relationships
disidentification, 49–50, *50*, 70, 72,
    93, *211*, 213
dissociating, 120
dominance and submission, 124, 143
dopamine, 9, 11, 131, *141*
dressing up, 3, 14, 154

Einstein, Albert, 70, 184, 212
ejaculatory control, 2, 19
Elders, Jocelyn, 133
embodiment. *See* health;
    interoception
emotion contagion, 64
emotional dynamics. *See* erotic
    cooperation
emotional sex, *141*, 142–43
emotional wounds. *See* erotic
    transformation; imprint
    portfolios; legacy states;
    planting hearts; shame; trauma;
    triggers; vulnerability

enchantment. *See* stage 1 relationships

*Enduring Desire,* 192

energy, 164. *See also* eros energy

erectile dysfunction, 24, 29, 38, 185, 187, 196, 199, 200

Ericsson, K. Anders, 165–66

EROS cycle, 173–83, 174, 205
  example of, 185–88
  exercise on, 188

eros energy, 146, 164, 223
  barriers to accessing, 13, 16, 177
  both/and approach and, 6
  creativity and, 34, 131, 171–72,
  as cyclical, 191, 194–95, 196
  four flavors of, 140–46, 141
  as gender bending, 154
  mindfulness and, 3, 14–15, 46–47, 169–73, 178–80
  mystery of, 45, 136, 162, 189, 214
  safety and, 130, 207
  sensuality and, 210

erotica, 14

erotic alchemy, 212–15

erotic attunement, 7, 47, 50, 85, 161–88, 211, 223
  EROS cycle and, 173–83, 174
  example of, 185–87
  exercises on, 163, 177, 188
  as improvisational, 162–67, 170–71, 173, 176
  mindfulness and, 163, 165, 168, 169–73
  missteps during, 184–85
  plane of possibility and, 167–69, 168
  *See also* interoception

erotic cooperation, 7, 61–94, 194
  developing, 74–89, 206

exercises on, 65, 89–94
healing via, 102–25
lack of, 61–74

erotic dates, 204–5, 216

erotic emergence, 172

erotic expansion, 146–47, 147, 202

erotic expression, 7, 120–60, 173
  developing, 138–47
  examples of, 147–54
  exercises on, 155–60
  lack of, 129–37
  two dimensions of, 129, 145

erotic presence, 6, 33–60
  exercises on, 39–40, 56–60
  lack of, 33–37, 38–40, 50–51, 53–54
  mindfulness for, 37–38, 40–60

erotic sustenance, 7, 189–216
  abstinence and, 194–95
  couple work of, 193–94, 200–209
  exercises on, 209, 215–16
  health and, 195–99
  solo work of, 195–97, 202, 209–12

erotic transformation, 7, 95–128
  exercises on, 108–9, 126–28
  tools for, 102–14, 116–23
  wounds in need of, 95–102, 114–16, 123–25

estrogen, 197

evolutionary biology, 11, 18, 117, 208

exercise, 195–97

extended orgasm techniques, 2, 19

familiarity trance, 28, 33–38, 40
  overcoming, 42, 53–60

family dynamics. *See* imprint portfolios; legacy states; parenting

fantasies, 14, 30, 143

disturbing, 148–49

lack of, 154

routine, 161–62, 171, 186

*See also* parts play

fear, 67–70, 76, 201. *See also* vulnerability: fear of

feedback, 80, 85, 99, 107, 122, 181, 182

felt sense. *See* interoception

feminism, 103, 148

*Fifty Shades of Grey*, 143

fight-flight-freeze, 69, 118–19, 238n38

Fishbane, Mona, 67, 68, 84

five Ss, 114, 115. *See also* stop-study-share

foreplay, 4

Fraser, Cheryl, 203

Freud, Sigmund, 164

fun dates, 203–4, 216

gender, 103, 142, 200, 217

queering, 30, 124, 135, 154–55

genital prime, sexual prime vs., 198

genitals, health of, 196

Gibran, Kahlil, 22, 208

Gilbert, Elizabeth, 72

*Girls and Sex*, 38

goal-free sex, 12, 15, 24–25, 34, 37, 44, 199–201, 205

aging and, 190, 200

in EROS cycle, 173, 175, 178–79, 181–82, 183

exercises on, 30–32, 39–40

trauma and, 115–16, 117

goal-oriented sex. *See* orgasm-centered sex; performance trance

Goleman, Daniel, 77

Golson, Benny, 164

good sex, definitions of, 190, 200–201

Gordon, Kerry, 171

Greenspan, Miriam, 22

Grey Trend, 143

grief, 21–22, 42, 79, 106, 123

guilt, 30, 99, 101, 106, 117, 123, 181

shame vs., 132–33

habits. *See* automaticity

Hakomi Mindful Somatic Psychotherapy, 4, 56, 218, 234n53

healing, 5, 7, 19, 29–30, 102–28, 217

health, 1, 24, 47, 61, 68, 204

sexual, 190, 195–99

Healy, Tara, 42

*Heart and Soul of Sex, The*, 214

hidden factors, 26, 29, 96, 96–102, 165, 183

Hock, Dee, 15

Hormones. *See* biochemistry

*How to Change Your Mind*, 212

Hsin Hsin Ming, 45

humility, 56, 57, 58

hysterectomy, 196, 197

Iasenza, Suzanne, 134, 154

impermanence, 43, 45–46

imprint portfolios, 223

hidden factors in, 96–103, 111–12

mindful awareness of, 48–49, 193–94

sex-negative, 4, 6, 29, 96

*See also* legacy states; shame; trauma; triggers

improvisation, 162–67, 170–71, 173, 176

impulses, opening to, 52, 173, 175, 179–80, 211

instinctual sex, *141*, 141–42
intention vs. impact, 85
intercourse, alternatives to, 200–201
Internal Family Systems, 139, 218–19
internal models, 6, 56, 97–99,
    166, 188
interoception, 47–48, 163, 169–70, 223
    during conflict, 63, 75
    in EROS cycle, 7, 173, 174–75,
    176–77
    examples of, 99, 106, 120
    via somatic self-attunement, 102,
    109, 116–18, 125
    yoga and, 197

jade eggs, 196
Johanson, Greg, 56
Johnson, Sue, 208
Jung, C. J., 114

Kegan, Robert, 12
Kegels, 196
Kerner, Ian, 154, 200
kink, 2, 30, 49, 52, 134, 143
Klein, Marty, 184, 190, 198, 200
Kleinplatz, Peggy, 162

Langer, Ellen, 46, 170
Lao Tzu, 89, 161
Lazar, Sara, 47
Lee, Martha, 178
legacy states, 64–65, 134, 223
    exercises on, 89–94
    moving beyond, 74–89
    in reciprocal interaction loops,
    65–74
    *See also* imprint portfolios;
    planting hearts; trauma;
    vulnerability

libido, 164
    conflicting levels of, 61, 66
    low, 13, 18, 185, 190, 199
    *See also* arousal; eros energy
life force, 164
lifestyle diseases, 196
Lois, George, 171
longing, 208–9
*Love and War in Intimate
    Relationships*, 68, 73
love state, 11, 17, 33
*Loving with the Brain in Mind*, 68
Luskin, Fred, 85
Lyons, Marlena S., 78, 82, 135, 217

masculinity, 142, 195, 200
mastery, 166
masturbation, 141, 146–47, 155–56,
    196, 210
    during partner sex, 106, 201
    as taboo, 113–14, 133
mature love. *See* stage 3
    relationships
McCarthy, Barry, 51, 192–93, 200
memory, 100, 112
    *See also* black light syndrome;
    imprint portfolios; legacy states;
    planting hearts
Meditation. *See* mindfulness
Mencken, H. L., 9
menopause, 24, 106–7, 185, 196, 197
metta meditation, 80–81
Metz, Michael, 192–93, 200
mind/body dualism, 176–77
mindful coinvestigation, 86–89,
    211, 223
    commitment to, 102, 202, 206
    examples of, 104–7, 109, 111–12,
    118–23, 181–82

exercise on, 94
knowing when to stop, 111,
 119, 159
in parts play, 152
mindfulness, 3, 40–43, 210–12, 211
 benefits of, 77, 86, 170, 213–24
 disidentification and, 49–50, 50,
 70, 72, 93, 211, 213
 interconnection and, 81
 perfection vs., 165
 practices, 77, 80–81, 175, 197
 rules vs., 117–18
 solo practice of, 202
mindful self-study, 48–50, 52, 202,
 206, 210, 211, 224
 during conflict, 78–79, 83, 92
 in EROS cycle, 173, 174–75, 176–77,
 180, 181
 exercise on, 79, 126–27
 in parts play, 146, 150, 152, 155–57
 of triggers, 102–26, 193–94
 See also interoception
mindful sex, 2–3, 37–38, 40–60,
 204–206, 210–15, 211, 224
 acceptance and, 66
 beyond the body, 48–49
 as compassionate, 20–21
 disidentification and, 49–50, 50
 as embodied, 43, 47–48, 176–77,
 200–201
 using EROS cycle, 173–83
 for erotic transformation, 7,
 95–128
 exercises on, 56–60
 fantasies and, 155–58
 five features of, 43–48
 meditation before, 204, 210
 novelty and, 43, 46–47, 54–60
 novelty trap vs., 2–3, 14–15, 37

stopping during, 108–10
 See also erotic attunement; erotic
 collaboration; goal-free sex
mindful touch exercise, 58–60
monogamy, 18
 monogamish vs., 13, 153, 161
Morin, Jack, 148
music, mindfulness and, 170

naked path, 10–11, 21–22, 43, 74, 224
 care cycle, 81–86, 83
 EROS cycle, 173–83, 174, 188
 five Ss, 107–10, 114, 115
 mindful coinvestigation, 86–89
 parts play, 138–60, 205
 passion pyramid, 140–46, 141
 planting a heart, 112–14, 115
 PREP process, 75–82, 76
 response-agility, 102, 183–84
 reveal-reach-repair, 81–86, 83
 seeing fresh, 36–37, 56–58
 somatic self-attunement, 102,
 116–20
 See also mindful self-study;
 mindful sex
Neff, Kristin, 80
negativity cycle. See reciprocal
 interaction loops
Negoski, Emily, 207
nervous system
 arousal and, 13, 197
 conflict and, 68, 69, 76
 mindfulness and, 47, 77
neuroception, 68
neuroscience, 4, 68–70, 99–100, 101
 on neuroplasticity, 112, 120
 on perception, 35, 47, 102, 170,
 213–14
Nin, Anaïs, 20, 23, 130, 131, 137, 140

"no mistakes" policy, 137, 167, 179, 184, 202
nonattachment, 45–46
non-consensual sex. *See* trauma
non-monogamy, consensual, 13, 18, 153, 161
novelty state, *193, 194, 211, 212,* 224
  attunement and, 168, 169, 172
  deep vs. wide, 14
  mindfulness and, 3, 43, 46–47, 54–60, *211*
  *See also* seeing fresh
novelty trap, 2–3, 13–15, 18, 28
  mindfulness vs., 37, 50–53
  *See also* performance trance

objectification, 141
Ogden, Gina, 214, 219
oral sex, 201, 205
  as routine, 33, 149, 161, 186
  as taboo, 98, 133, 181
Orenstein, Peggy, 38
orgasm-centered sex, 18, 33–34, 39, 101. *See also* goal-free sex
orgasms, 45, 47, 196, 200, 207, 214
  lack of, 29, 181, 197, 198
oxytocin, 11, 13, *141, 142,* 207–208

pain points, 23–24, 25. *See also* triggers
parenting, 85, 151
  as barrier to sex, 1, 33, 54, 191, 194, 207
parts play, 138–60, 205, 224
  context for, 149, 154, 155, 159
  examples of, 147–53
  exercises on, 155–60
  masturbatory fantasy and, 146–47
  passion pyramid and, 140–46

Passion and Presence retreats, 1–4, 65, 225*n*1. *See also* case studies
passion pyramid, 140–46, *141,* 158, 204
pelvic floor exercises, 196
penetration, alternatives to, 200–201
PEP. *See* pure erotic potential
perception, 27–28, 35–36, 41
  mindfulness and, 49–50, 55, 212–15
  *See also* seeing fresh
Perel, Esther, 143, 208, 219
perennial wisdom, 22, 43
performance anxiety, 95–96, 107, 185, 200
performance trance, 28, 29, 38, 101, 117, 190, 218
  erotic attunement vs., 163–66, *165,* 171, 173, 175, 178–79, 183
  as novelty trap, 2–3, 13–15, 18, 37
  parts play vs., 139, 140
  waking up from, 50–53, 199–201
personal growth, 23–24, 25, 28, 40, 73–74, 183–84, 192–93, 202, 206
  inhibiting of, 62, 97, 137, 193
  *See also* stage 3 relationships
physical sex, 141, 141–42
plane of possibility, 168–69, *169,* 178
planting hearts, 107, 112–14, *115,* 194, 224
  exercises on, 127–28, 205
  to overcome shame, 135, 150–51, 152
  to overcome trauma, 116, 119–22, 125, 238*n*38
pleasure, 47–48, 117–18
  diverse pathways to, 42, 45–46, 50, 116, 200–201, 214
  exercises on, 58–60, 210
  guilt about, 98–99, 131, 217
  receiving vs. giving, 110, 141–42

savoring, 173, *174*, 175, 180–83

signaling, 181

speed and, 12

Pollan, Michael, 212, 213

Porges, Stephan, 69, 208

porn, 14, 153

power dynamics, 48, 67, 78, 87, 143, 148–49

pranayama, 197

predictive coding, 212. *See also* perspective; trances

pregnancy, unwanted, 200, 207

PREP process, 75–82, *76*, 158

prostate cancer, 196, 199, 245*n*26

protective strategies, 62, 64–65, 67–72

  in defend cycle, 103, *104*, 109

  exercises on, 65, 89–94

  exploring, 74–85

  mindful coinvestigation of, 86–89, 94, 120

  in parts play, 151–53

Psaris, Jett, 78, 82, 135, 217

psychological sex, *141*, 143, 149

puberty, 141, 150

*pudendum*, etymology of, 133

pure erotic potential (PEP), 15–16, 170, 224

  barriers to, 24–30, *27*, 62, 96, 130, 165, 183, 207 (*see also specific barriers*)

  in EROS cycle, 173–74, *174*

  growth and, 23–25, *25*

  mindfulness and, 40–50, 212–15

  plane of possibility and, 168–69, *169*

  state of mind and, 39–40, 115

  *See also* mindful sex; naked path; stage 3 relationships

queerness, 11, 78, 98, 124–25, 134–35, 154

race, 78, 98

radical nakedness, 83–84, 224. *See also* naked path; vulnerability

Real, Terrence, 142

reciprocal interaction loops (RIL), 70–72, *71*, 218, 224

  example of, 66–67

  interrupting, 74–89

  diagramming of, *71*, 89–94

re-enchantment. *See* stage 3 relationships

relationships, 72–74, 201–8

  conflict in, 61–74

  cooperation in, 74–94, 206, 217

  covenants in, 201–202

  divergent fantasies in, 144, 145–55

  making time for, 203–5

  satisfaction in, 195, 203

  sexless, 1, 2, 12, 185, 191, 194–95, 196

  three-stage model of, 11–23, *193*

  *See also* erotic cooperation; stage 1 relationships; stage 2 relationships; stage 3 relationships

resilience practices, 77, 80–81, 175, 197

response-agility, 102, 159, 173, 178–79, 183–84, 218, 236*n*21

  for healing, 116, 118–19, 128, 194

  reasons for, 183

  in stop-study-share, 107–10

retreats, self-guided, 203, 215

reveal-reach-repair, 81–86, *83*, 157

RIL. *See* reciprocal interaction loops

Rilke, Rainer Maria, 65
risk, fear of. *See* safety trance
Robins, Tom, 189
Rogers, Carl, 62
role-play, 14, 83, 138, 143, 161–62, 171.
    *See also* parts play
romance culture, 21, 28, 73, 84
Rumi, 64, 103

sadomasochism, 143
safety trance, 28, 130, 131, 132, 135–37
    animal instincts vs., 142
    overcoming, 138–40
    racy version of, 161–62, 171
safety zone, 136, 137, 206–208
    expansion of, 146, 146–47, 202
safe words, 109, 159, 205
Sapolsky, Robert, 76
Savage, Dan, 13
schemas, 98–99
Schnarch, David, 107, 145, 192, 198, 219
Schwartz, Richard, 139, 151, 218–19
seeing fresh, 36–37, 54–56, 167, 202,
    203, 211, 212, 224
    exercises on, 56–58
self-esteem, 132–33, 197–98
    self-compassion vs., 80–81
self-regulation, 70, 77, 211
    via disidentification, 49–50, 50,
    70, 72, 93, 211, 213
self-study. *See* mindful self-study
selves, as multidimensional, 62–65,
    129–31, 136, 137–38, 172
    naming, 71, 72, 90, 91–92, 129, 144,
    146, 149, 150, 152, 158
    *See also* parts play
Sengstan, 45
sex, 200–201, 204–6
    aspects of, 110

change and, 15, 190, 212, 214
darker side of, 97
dissatisfaction with, 2, 16–19
health benefits of, 194, 196
initiating, 48, 99, 110, 124,
    179–80, 202
legality of, 133
motivations for, 39, 140–46, *141*
relationship satisfaction and, 195,
    203
*See also* mindful sex
sex therapy, 3, 4, 214. *See also* case
    studies
sex toys, 3, 14, 133, 187, 199, 201
sexual abuse, 47, 116–24, 142, 197. *See
    also* trauma
sexual concordance, 47–48
sexual excitatory system, 207
sexual inhibitory system, 207
*Sexual Intelligence*, 184
sexual orientation, 11, 78, 98,
    134–35, 200
sexual positions, 3, 14, 37, 190
sexual skills. *See* performance trance
sexual warriors, 2–3, 28, 38, 50–53. *See
    also* performance trance
sex workers, 141
Shakespeare, William, 16
shame, 100, 109–10, 131–35
    as barrier to PEP, 26, 29, 30, 130, 183
    examples of, 19, 49, 95, 103–7,
    111–12, 151
    guilt vs., 132–33
    overcoming, 4, 7, 138–60, 179–80
Sheinkman, Michele, 67, 84
Siegel, Dan, 168, 169, 233$n$44
Solomon, Marion, 68, 73
somatic psychology. *See* body-
    centered psychotherapy

somatic self-attunement, 102, 109, 116–18, 125, 163, 176–77, 224. *See also* interoception

soul mates, 72–74

spirituality, 22, 199

spiritual sex, *141*, 144, 149

stage 1 relationships, 6, 9, 11–16, 25, 84, 191, *193*

awareness during, 35, 55

biochemistry of, 11, 33, 97, 101

expansiveness during, 20, 61

length of, 5, 101

selves in, 130, 134

trying to recreate, 40, 45, 203

stage 2 relationships, 1–30, 191–92, *193*, 203

abstinence in, 1, 2, 12, 185

biochemistry of, 13

conflict in, 61–74

crises and, 23–24

as goal-oriented, 12, 15, 24–25

hidden factors appearance during, 97, 101–2, 133–34

incompatibility and, 2, 4, 17, 24, 28–29, 66

inevitability of, 6, 9–10, 11–12, 16

novelty trap and, 2–3, 13–15, 28

outside attraction in, 23–24, 35, 36, 37, 137, 153

PEP-limiting mind-sets in, 24–30, *27*, *62*, *64*, *96*, *130*, *165*, *183*, 207 (*see also specific barriers*)

physical changes and, 1, 24, 38, 106–7

prevalence of, 2

as routine, 1, 6–7, 13, 17, 18, 23, 27, 28, 33–38, 40, 131, 136, 145, 161–62, 167–68, 183, 213

stress and, 1, 12–13, 33, 61, 130, 203

typecasting in, 129–31, 203

unspoken agreements in, 136

stage 3 relationships, 6–7, 20–23, 192, *193*, 224

abstinence in, 191, 194–95, 196

cooperation in, 74–85

conscious contracts in, 137–38, 153, 201–2

dates in, 202–6

full selves in, 10, 64, 131, 137–60

grief and, 21–22

healing in, 5, 7, 19, 29–30, 107–25

improvisation in, 162–63

mindfulness in, 43–50, 210–15

no mistakes policy in, 137, 167, 179, 184, 202

solo work of, 79, 195–97, 202, 209–12

space in, 10, 208–9

whole body sex in, 200–201

willingness in, 194, 204

*See also* erotic sustenance; mindful sex; naked path; pure erotic potential; response-agility

state-dependent memory, 97, 101–102

stop signals, 109, 159, 205

stop-study-share, 107–10, 114, 115, 127, 157, 205

Stosney, Steven, 41

stretching, 163, 177

sustenance plans, 215–16

Tantra, 2

*Tao Te Ching*, 161

Taoism, 5, 89, 161

Tatkin, Stan, 68, 73, 76, 77

tending dates, 205, 215–16

testosterone, 11, 13, 199

therapy, 73
  body-centered, 4, 5, 164, 177, 218,
    219, 238*n*36, 238*n*38–39
  couples, 67
therapy
  sex, 3, 4, 214
  trauma, 4, 116, 218, 219, 238*n*36
  *See also* case studies
three Rs (reveal, reach, and repair),
  81–86, 83, 157
threesomes, 161
trances, 26, 27–28, 183, 208, 212,
  218, 224
  mindfulness as antidote to, 41,
    49–56
  *See also* familiarity trance;
    performance trance; safety
    trance
trauma, 2, 100, 114–25
  as barrier to PEP, 16, 26, 30–31
  embodiment and, 117–19, 177
  healing from, 5, 7, 116–25, 238*n*38
  partners of survivors of, 123–25
  reactivity and, 69–70, 76, 85
  secondary, 115–16
  sociocultural, 78
  therapy for, 4, 116, 218, 219,
    238*n*36
  *See also* black light syndrome;
    imprint portfolios; legacy states;
    planting a heart
triggers, 5, 7, 19, 29, 193, 211
  addressing, 75–89, 103–14, 104, 105,
    194, 202, 218
  avoiding partners', 123–25, 131, 136,
    137, 156

common pain points as, 23–24, 25
emotional, 61, 64–72, 95–128, 162
Tronic, Ed, 184
turn-offs, 144, 145–46, 207

unwanted touch. *See* trauma

vagal nerves, 69, 75, 77, 207
vasopressin, 13, *141*
Ventura, Michael, 153–54, 214
vulnerability, 7, 10
  cycle of, 67–89, *71, 83,* 151–53
  in EROS cycle, 174, 179–80
  exercises on, 89–94
  fear of, 26, 28–29, 30–31, 62, 64–65,
    75, 99, 134, 183
  of partners, 84, 123–25, 136, 194
  revealing of, 82–83, 201

Wald, Lana, 51
Weiss, Halko, 4, 70, 72, 78, 218, 220–21
  diagrams developed by, *50, 90*
Welwood, John, 30, 62, 74, 82, 166,
  170, 210, 217–18
  on vulnerability, 21, 61, 82
whole-body sex, 200–201
whole-person multimodal sex, 131,
  138–40, 146–47, 153–55, 172. *See
  also* erotic expression
wounds, unhealed. *See* erotic
  transformation; imprint
  portfolios; legacy states;
  planting hearts; shame; trauma;
  triggers; vulnerability

yoga, 177, 197

# About the Author

Maci Daye is an AASECT Certified Sex Therapist, Licensed Professional Counselor, and Certified Therapist and Trainer of Hakomi Mindful Somatic Psychotherapy. As a sex therapist, her focus is on helping couples deepen their erotic connection mindfully. Maci has been leading *Passion & Presence*® couples retreats and professional workshops in the USA, Europe, Mexico, Australia, and New Zealand since 2010. A frequent conference presenter, Maci has graduate degrees from Harvard Univerwsity and Georgia State University. She also completed the Level 2 Somatic Experiencing trauma training developed by Peter Levine. To learn more about her programs or to contact Maci go to www.passionandpresence.com.